THE
Emotional Energy
FACTOR

The Secrets
High-Energy People Use
to Beat Emotional Fatigue

Mira Kirshenbaum

DELTA TRADE PAPERBACKS

THE EMOTIONAL ENERGY FACTOR
A Delta Book

PUBLISHING HISTORY
Delacorte Press hardcover edition published January 2003
Delta trade paperback edition / January 2004

Published by
Bantam Dell
A Division of Random House, Inc.
New York, New York

ISBN 0-440-50925-4

Manufactured in the United States of America
Published simultaneously in Canada

BVG
10 9 8 7 6 5 4 3 2 1

Praise for
The Emotional Energy Factor

"In this upbeat and consumer-friendly how-to ... Kirshenbaum helps readers identify the roots of their lethargy, and implement the appropriate strategies for regaining their spunk. Her solutions are straightforward . . . it may be enough to lift readers out of the doldrums." —*Publishers Weekly*

"Fascinating! I think people need to grasp the premise in this book that physical energy amounts to only thirty percent of total energy. Seventy percent of a person's energy must come from emotional energy. Everyone should read this book. Thyroid patients could especially be empowered with such knowledge."
  —Kelly R. Hale, President, American Foundation of Thyroid Patients

"Kirshenbaum offers concrete tips for increasing emotional energy, peppering her advice with real-life anecdotes." —*Dayton Daily News* (Ohio)

"Every woman I know needs the sound, simple, and satisfying advice Mira Kirshenbaum so effectively offers here. Read this life-changing book, and you'll not only release the negative emotions that are paralyzing your life— you'll also reclaim the positive energy necessary to add more joy to your days and vitality to your years. I highly recommend it!"
  —Debra Waterhouse, M.P.H., R.D., author of *Outsmarting Female Fatigue*

"Mira Kirshenbaum's latest book addresses the most important and least understood ingredient in maintaining high energy. This practical, easy-to-understand book takes cutting-edge research and puts it in the hands and hearts of everyone who wants the opportunity for a high-spirited life. Every patient I see asks me how to increase energy; Mira has provided the answer. Highly recommended."
  —Arthur P. Ciaramicoli, Ed.D., Ph.D., author of *The Power of Empathy*

"Mira Kirshenbaum's book brims over with emotional energy, providing clear access to the rich resources we all carry within us. . . . I recommend this book to all of us who tend to feel deeply depleted by the demands and stresses of our busy lives."
  —Rabbi Ted Falcon, Ph.D., author of *A Journey of Awakening*

To the countless people who have given me
so much emotional energy over the years
by reaching out with letters, phone calls, and e-mails
to tell me how much my books have helped them

ACKNOWLEDGMENTS

You can do what I did. You can even make a game of it. Think about all the people in your life, everyone you know, and guess which ones have emotional energy.

It's not always easy to tell. Some very quiet people are filled with it. Some very perky, positive-sounding people are putting up a brave front and really have little emotional energy.

Everyone who reads this book will be able to tell who is who. But once you sense who has emotional energy, then those people have a real gift for you. Emotional energy is contagious. When you're with someone who has it, you start feeling it too.

People with emotional energy also have a special gift for me. These are the people that I most want to thank for making this book possible. They are friends, colleagues, teachers, students, clients, acquaintances, and family. They are also wonderful strangers who agreed to participate in the research much of this book is based on. Each of them taught me important lessons about how we lose emotional energy and what we can do to get it back.

I can't thank everyone by name. There are just too many. But I must single out Herbert Berghof, Ruth Bork, Diane Boudreau, Martin Buber, Judith Chan, Lynette Cunningham, Mihaly Csikszentmihalyi, Norma de Jesus, Marybeth English, Nancy Fain, Esther Feiler, Roger Fisher, Sonia Freund, Vivian Green, Shere Hite, Kathleen Huntington, Alfred Kazin, Allan Kaprow, Pearl Karch, Carolyn Kreinsen, Rabbi Harold Kushner, Matt Lauer, Chloe Madanes, Franny Peterson, Sally Jessy Raphael, Father Bill Richardson, Cynthia Roe, Naomi Saperstein, Virginia Satir, Pepper Schwartz, Sallie Sears, Gitta Sereny, Pilani Shipp, Isaac Bashevis Singer, Patti Smith, John Stossel, DeeDee Warren, Rosa Wexler, Carl Whitaker, and Elie Wiesel.

It's an open secret that my partner and husband, Dr. Charles Foster, and I are full, 50/50 collaborators on all of our books. This book was no exception. Every word, every idea, is as much his as it is mine. For years we worked on the research together, trying to pinpoint exactly what it is that people do to get more emotional energy for themselves. Those writers who work in utter solitude—how do they do it? Without the energy Charles has brought to this process, I don't know if this book would have been possible.

I feel very lucky to have the best agent in the business, Howard Morhaim. Our relationship is eight years old now, a long one in publishing, I think. Howard's been great to me through all my ups and downs, and I'm very thankful.

I'm also lucky to have a terrific editor, Danielle Perez, who believes in me and deeply understands what I'm trying to do. Danielle immediately had the vision to see what was important about this project. And she worked brilliantly to make sure that the final book lived up to that vision.

Barb Burg has the reputation of being one of the smartest publicity people in publishing, and I'm grateful for everything she and all the other wonderful people in her department have done to bring this book to people's attention.

After working on eight books, I can say that my copy editor, Sue Warga, is the best I've ever had.

This book is filled with people. My last and greatest debt is to the men and women who shared their lives with me. Their stories of emotional fatigue and emotional energy, in their own words, are a deep source of inspiration and understanding. You know who you are, and I thank you with all my heart.

CONTENTS

TO MY READER

Welcome to the energy revolution. This book introduces a radical new approach to getting the kind of energy we'd all like. It's based on the discovery that feeling energetic comes from having physical energy and having emotional energy, but for most of us today it's emotional energy that's in shortest supply. If you're looking for more energy, it's overwhelmingly likely that what you need is more emotional energy.

In these pages you'll discover just what emotional energy is and why it's so important. Most of all, you'll discover exactly what you can do to tap into the reserves of emotional energy that already exist within you.

This book is filled with the kind of help I like to get, the way I like to get it. I don't like simplistic, one-size-fits-all solutions, and I bet you don't either. Instead, the help you'll find here is based on what works for real people living with the daily pressures we all face. And it's respectful of our individuality. These pages will show you how to unlock your emotional energy and experience your own personal energy revolution.

Please visit *www.emotionalenergyfactor.com*. Let's keep in touch.

THE
Emotional
Energy
FACTOR

So—How's Your Emotional Energy?

If you've been looking for more energy, you're not alone. Millions of people every day confess things like "I wish I had more energy." "I just can't get started in the morning." "Thinking about the long busy day ahead makes me feel overwhelmed." "There are things I want to do, and I know I'll enjoy doing them, but I find myself saying no to them instead of yes." "I'm just feeling so drained, tense, glum these days." "What I hate about not having energy is the way it makes me feel older than I am." "Where's the fun I was looking forward to in my life?"

You don't need a reason for wanting more energy—you just know you need more. But many of us can point to special reasons why we need more.

Sometimes our energy is under attack because we're going through a major life transition. Change is exhausting. And it's not just negative changes such as going through a divorce or dealing with a loved one's illness that deplete our energy. Positive changes too—getting married, starting a new job, or having a baby—take a lot out of us.

Sometimes our energy gets depleted because of a medical condition.

1

Any illness from a bad cold on up can make a person feel drained. And some illnesses specifically attack a person's natural energy level. If there's something wrong with your body, you need more energy now.

Sometimes we want more energy even though we're young: "I'm only twenty-four, and it just feels nuts for me to be so tired." Or we want more energy because we're getting older: "As I'm getting up in years, energy is the one thing I need more than anything else, now more than ever."

And sometimes we want more energy because our plates are just so damned full, and after a while it starts to get to us. "It's not just that there's so much for me to do every day, and so much to think about. That takes enough pushing. But then I have to do a really bang-up job too."

But we all understand how important energy is. We understand that the biggest difference between people who get what they want out of life and people who don't is *energy*. You could be the smartest, most attractive, most talented person in the world, but without energy you'd go nowhere, like a meatball that's fallen on the floor.

With energy everything is possible. It's energy that gives life its sweetness and tang. It's energy that makes you feel like you. It's energy that makes your dreams come true.

So—how's *your* energy? If you're like most of us, you want and need more. Well, you've come to the right place. This book will show you why you've been losing energy and what to do to get all the energy you want.

Where to Find Your Missing Energy

I know you've already tried to get more energy from many sources. But I'll bet they've mostly been sources of physical energy, like PowerBars and coffee, exercise and vitamins. And these haven't been enough.

Gail, 29: "Where's my get up and go? I was on the soccer team in high school and college. Track too. I always take care of myself. I eat right, I live right. Eight hours' sleep and I'd wake up fully refreshed, ready to go out and have fun. Now I'm still doing all the same things. The doctor said

I'm fine physically. So why am I tired all the time? But it's not my body that's tired. It's like it's *me* that's tired inside my body."

Millions of us feel the way Gail feels.* The problem is that if you're like most Americans, you're close to being maxed out on the amount of additional energy you can get from physical sources. Physical energy sources are anything you go to for your body's energy needs, everything from food and rest to a carefully thought out exercise program and a full complement of vitamins. And sure, maybe you could get more sleep or eat a little more healthfully, but the truth is that people living in the developed world today are healthier and more vital than ever before. If you're feeling you need more energy, the problem is most likely not with your body.

No wonder so many of us are caught in an energy rat race. The more we need energy, the more we try to boost our physical energy, but we don't get the pop we're looking for because there's not much more to get from physical sources. We search for still newer sources of physical energy anyway, and they don't help much either.

Now you see why it's been so hard to find more energy. You're looking in the wrong place.

Emotional Energy Is the Answer

You're not just a body, are you? So it's not just your body that needs more energy. It's you, a whole person. You know that the emotional side of you is as important as your body. So it makes sense that there's another energy source. It's *emotional energy*.

Emotional energy is the kind of energy you're looking for anyway. It's not an adrenaline-filled, run-around-like-a-nut kind of energy where you burn too brightly. It's a special energy that's all about feeling young and

---

*To protect people's privacy and ensure that they would open up to me, I promised everyone I interviewed that I would change his or her name, as well as all identifying details.

deeply connected to the fun and hope in life. Everyone's experienced a moment when the chips were down and all you saw ahead was a tough, uphill climb, and yet you felt full of vitality. That's emotional energy—an aliveness of the mind, a happiness of the heart, and a spirit filled with hope. How could you possibly feel energetic unless you had that kind of energy?

Isn't this what we all want: an energetic mind and heart and soul in an energetic body? I call it complete energy:

Complete energy = physical energy + emotional energy

We now know that the physical side is actually the less important part. I asked energy experts such as endocrinologists, nutritionists, and specialists in sports medicine, "How much energy does the typical American get from physical sources and how much from emotional ones?" When I averaged out their answers, I was stunned. Physical energy can supply at most 30 percent of your total energy. Even if you had perfect physical health and ate the perfect diet and got the perfect amount of exercise, all that would give you only 30 percent of the complete energy you need.* The remaining 70 percent of the energy you need must come from your emotional energy. And you need a lot.

Where I First Saw That Emotional Energy Matters

Let's face it, life is designed to exhaust our emotional energy. Most of us work damned hard. We have obligations to our family and friends. We join organizations. We have dreams and ambitions we push ourselves to achieve. Sometimes just when we think we're stretched to the limit, some

---

*If you're wondering whether you could do more to address your body's needs for physical energy, check out the Appendix, "The *Physical* Energy Factor."

disaster or emergency stretches us even further. A family member gets sick. We get laid off. Someone we love dumps us. A pet project fails. One step forward, two steps back.

And yet we all know people filled with verve and joy in spite of all this. That's the difference emotional energy makes.

I think you have to see people thriving in spite of difficult circumstances to really appreciate it. I started seeing this when I was a kid, and it's always stayed with me.

I grew up poor in New York City. My mother and I were refugees from Europe. She started out working in a garment factory twelve hours a day. Everyone in our neighborhood was an immigrant. Everyone had it tough. Life could really get to people. But if our world was a constant struggle to find work, pay the rent, educate the children, and afford clothes you weren't ashamed to wear, people reacted to it very differently. Some were so exhausted they gave up trying. Some kept on pushing, but that's all it was—pushing. They were running on empty. You saw it in their self-pity, their rage, their constant anxiety, their utter discouragement. You saw it in their burned-out eyes, like soldiers who've spent too many days in combat.

So are we fools to wish we had more energy? Should we all just declare the human condition permanently pooped?

No! Growing up I also saw people who in spite of everything were filled with a special kind of inner energy. They led the same lives as everyone else. But still they had hopes and dreams. Still they made good things happen. Still they found ways to make themselves happy and stay upbeat.

My Uncle Morris was like this. He worked long hours managing a laundry. His wife was a crazy troublemaker—everyone said so. His kids were no bargains. Everything in his life was a struggle. But he was always emotionally vibrant. He kept working on plans for owning his own business. He was always taking us on trips to the country. He was always singing and teaching us new songs. And whenever he visited, he took the trouble to bring a box of candy or cookies especially for me.

High-Energy People Have High *Emotional* Energy

I'm sure you too know people who have plenty of energy no matter what, as if they'd found a secret stash. I'm talking about people who do a lot, are upbeat, and get a lot of enjoyment from what they do even though so many forces in life seem to be against them. But we don't think of them as living in an unattainable stratosphere. There's something about being filled with energy that makes us feel, "Yeah, I can see myself like that." We know intuitively that emotional energy is our birthright.

We wish we knew these people's secrets because of the enormous difference we know emotional energy makes in their lives. And that difference is the *emotional energy factor*.

- A man spends his life hanging in there, working at a job he doesn't like, struggling to support his family, and all the while he remains cheerful, never complaining. *Without emotional energy, this man would've become just another miserable, angry guy*.
- A young woman spends years trying to find herself, to figure out what work she wants to do and how she wants to live. It's confusing and it should be discouraging, but she hangs in there, full of hope, knowing that every person can find a life that fits. *Without emotional energy, this young woman would have given up*.
- A man spends years dealing with a chronic, debilitating physical condition and yet radiates warmth and hope: Instead of spreading gloom, he spreads joy. *Without emotional energy, he might've collapsed physically and become bitter, cold, and lonely*.
- It's Wimbledon. The deciding match of the men's finals. Two world-class tennis players have been going full out for hours. Both are in superb physical shape. But at this stage in a grueling competition that stretches the human soul to its limit, one player will keep on finding the fun in the game, will keep on wanting to win the most. *Without emotional energy, the winner would've been the loser*.

- Look at some of the greatest artists, producing beauty out of darkness, joy out of misery. There are many, like the painter Renoir, who was racked with pain from arthritis, almost unable to hold a brush in his hands, or Rembrandt, who struggled with loneliness and poverty. Yet both worked for years producing one radiant masterpiece after another. Then there were Beethoven and Mozart. Both of them produced some of their most shining, happy music during times when the circumstances of their lives were most desperate and filled with loss. Many great artists have had difficult lives. *Without emotional energy, think of all the great art that never would have been born.*

- A scientist or inventor faces years of heart- and spirit-breaking frustration and yet keeps on trying until he finally reaches the brass ring he's been struggling toward. *Without emotional energy, almost no difficult scientific or technological problem would have been solved.*

- An inner-city woman works at low-paying jobs and brings up six children, sending them all to college. And that's the easy part. The hard part is that all the while she inculcates in them a loving, hopeful spirit. *Without emotional energy, life would crush many of us.*

- Think about a person so passionate for a cause that he or she fights for it in spite of everything. Gandhi is an example—he spent long periods of time fasting, depriving his body of energy, yet finding an energy source that enabled him to fight the British Empire. *Without emotional energy, we'd all be stuck with every form of injustice.*

- Why has Anne Frank touched so many of us? It's not just because of what happened to her—similar stories happened to millions. But in spite of the most oppressive conditions, we can read from her own pen how she radiates a kind of hope and spunk. *Without emotional energy, the human spirit could not survive for long.*

The more pressures you have to deal with, the more important it is to take care of your emotional energy. As you can see, *it's the most precious form of energy you have*. It's the kind you need the most of. It's the kind that makes your life feel satisfying and enables you to do something with it.

Having Emotional Energy
Changes Everything

Every dimension of who you are feels better the more emotional energy you have. Let's start with your body. Suppose you've been working unusually hard. Long hours, not enough sleep, not enough healthy food.

Well, this is where emotional energy comes to the rescue. If there's a group at the office working this hard, those with the most emotional energy will feel the best and be able to keep on going the longest. This makes sense. Why do people poop out? It's not just physical exhaustion. The first ones to drop out are the ones who get discouraged and feel most emotionally drained.

Emotional energy comes to the rescue when the body has reached its limits. In fact, I've seen people damaged by disease whose physical energy has been beaten into the ground but who are able to fight on because their emotional energy gives them the hum and spark they need.

Laura Hillenbrand wrote a best-selling book while in the midst of suffering from chronic fatigue syndrome. It was so bad that in interviews she talked about "my broken body." On her best days she had only enough physical energy to drag herself out of bed to write at her computer for an hour or two.

But ah! the miracle of emotional energy. She had a story she cared about. The joy of sharing it filled her with energy. The fun of playing with words and anecdotes gave her fuel. And so she wrote *Seabiscuit,* about an unlikely horse who became a champion. No one who reads this book could imagine it had been written by someone crippled by an extreme deprivation of physical energy. But that's the power of emotional energy.

I know about this from the inside. I'd been going along doing my work, but for about a year I'd noticed there was something wrong with me. I had to push myself to do everything I'd been doing easily before. I found myself sleeping more but feeling less refreshed. I had aches throughout my body, including my heart. I had no desire to exercise. Physically I felt more and more dragged down and clogged up.

Finally I went for a checkup. I'll never forget how the phone rang around midnight a few days later and woke me up out of a deep sleep. It was my doctor. The lab had just called her, waking her up. My thyroid levels were so low that it was an emergency. As my doctor said, "With levels this low I'm amazed that you're able to function."

Yet my spirits were up, and I'd been functioning fine, although I was in the worst physical state of my life. How could this be? This was precisely the period when I was doing research and learning secrets about what people do to get more energy. Emotional energy is such a powerful force that just hearing the secrets of high-energy people enabled me to keep going in spite of a condition that usually knocks people out of circulation.

Emotional energy can come to the rescue no matter what physical condition you're struggling with. Physical energy is limited under the best of circumstances. But your emotional energy is potentially unlimited. And unlike physical energy, which runs down as we get older, emotional energy can increase the more you learn what works best for you. Imagine that: every year of your life getting more and more energy.

Emotional energy can actually change your appearance. Let me ask you this—why are there two words, *beautiful* and *attractive*? Because they're different things. We've all seen beautiful people who seem dull and lifeless. We know they embody physical perfection, but we're not attracted to them. Maybe we think we should be, but we're not.

Yet someone can be attractive without being beautiful. When we say someone's attractive, we say we're drawn to them. There's a magnetism. They radiate light. Notice that these words have to do with energy. When we're drawn to someone, it's their energy that draws us. And it's the emotional energy factor that makes all the difference. People who look happy and alive arouse more attraction than blank but pretty faces. Imagine what more emotional energy will do for *your* appearance.

While looking good and feeling good are important, other things are as important. Like changing your life, if that's what you want to do. When you increase your emotional energy, it's amazing how your dreams become realities. And that's because obstacles lose the power to stop you.

Pick a dream, any dream. A couple starting out thinks it's impossible to save for a down payment on a house. But emotional energy makes it possible to hang in there and do what it takes to get that down payment.

You're stuck in a job you don't like and dream of launching a freelance career. It's emotional energy that keeps you focused and protects your hopes so you can get going and keep on going.

You're stuck in a troubled relationship. What else but emotional energy can make it possible for you to hang in there and make things better or develop the courage to get out when you see that nothing can be improved?

You've dreamed of completing your education. But there are so many demands on your time. Emotional energy makes it possible for you to say yes to yourself and no to others so you can make this dream come true.

There are countless stories of people whose dreams came true because they had more emotional energy. For now, here are just two.

Sara, 44: "Trying to get pregnant after 40 is not for sissies. The first in vitro we tried failed. I was devastated. I saw I was in for a long and difficult journey, and there was no guarantee I'd have a baby at the end. My emotional energy was at a very low level. Thank God I avoided making a mistake I think many women make. I didn't wait for a baby to make everything all right. I knew I had to get my energy in a good place. So I did everything I could to feel emotionally nourished. That made all the difference.

"Of course there were lots of difficulties. The hardest was a miscarriage after a couple of failed tries. Now that I have the daughter I've always wanted, I'm glad I hung in there. Without emotional energy I wouldn't have persisted. If I hadn't persisted, I wouldn't have my daughter now."

Don, 32: "I was actually one of the first of those dot-com start-up people. And we'd gotten pretty big too. But then there was the crash of

2000. Everyone reacted differently. Most people were shellshocked. But in spite of all the crap I had to deal with, I had a lot of emotional energy and we hung in there. Nothing had to be a certain way. Everything was flexible. Size didn't matter. So we survived. And we're gonna survive."

There's another word for making your dreams come true: *success*.

Here are some truths about success that make clear the huge role emotional energy plays. Success means having to deal with lots of rejection, frustration, difficulty, and defeat along the way. It means taking risks. And it means finding the strength to stay connected to what you really care about.

There are always two paths: an easy path that doesn't take much out of you but doesn't take you anywhere special, and a tough, scary path that takes you to where a dream comes true. This harder path places huge demands on your energy. The easy path lies in wait, tempting you to give up your dreams.

Now you see the risk. Low energy doesn't mean you'll find it harder to keep going. It means you'll fall off the path that leads to your success and end up on the path of least resistance which leads to Nowheresville. But don't worry. However drained you feel, you can get back your full energy.

How to Tell if You're Emotionally Fatigued

People *know* there's something wrong with their emotional energy. It may creep up on you, but then it hits you that emotionally your tires have gone flat. This can come at any time. Sometimes it comes after you've been struggling with a difficult situation for a long time.

Molly, 32: "People think of me as a dynamo. I'm always on the go, and I love being active. But I've been in this relationship for two years now, and it's just bad. We have nothing in common. We don't click. I know it's over. I have to end it. But two years of struggle and disappointment have left me so weak I don't have it in me to help myself. I know what I have to do, but I can't bring myself to do it. And the fact that this hasn't worked out somehow makes me feel disheartened about everything."

Sometimes the realization that you've lost emotional energy comes after you've had the rug pulled out from under you.

John, 36: "When so many of us got laid off, I thought, Okay, this is going to be tough, but I know the drill, so I'll work at finding a job and I'll be fine. It was hard because I'd had a future with that company and that's gone. But, you know, be a man. I get that. I mean, I'm a triathlete, for chrissake. But I don't feel any bounce in me. I go through the motions of job hunting, but I'm scared I'm not going to be able to keep going. It's easier to take just any job."

And sometimes, scarily enough, the realization comes out of nowhere.

Julia, 41: "I've always loved gardening. And I've had this garden for years that's been my pride and joy. Now it's March and I should be in a fever of excitement. But it's the most mysterious thing. I'm just not interested. My garden was everything to me. Now it feels like nothing. I mean, I know I'll do something, I always do—rake away dead leaves, whatever. But it's a chore now. What's happening? Where's my energy for this?"

Wherever it comes from, here's what emotional fatigue feels like. When you check in with yourself to see if there's any fizz left, you feel flat. Down. Blah. Glum. In a slump. Irritable. Too pooped to pop. Discouraged. Nervous. Out of ideas. Older than your years. Gripped by an inner fatigue that's hard to shake.

Is it the same as depression? That depends. A major depression is a life-threatening psychiatric disorder that needs professional attention. You know you're suffering from a major depression if you're paralyzed with emotional pain and unable to function in your life. When you see someone with major depression, it's very striking. Anyone suffering from it should make getting treatment the top priority.

On the other hand, most of the time when people talk about being depressed they are talking about emotional exhaustion to one degree or another. For these people—and these are the vast majority of people to whom the word *depression* is casually applied—the fastest, most effective, and most healthful treatment isn't getting a prescription or finding out how you really feel about your mother. Instead, it's finding specific things to do to build up your emotional energy.

Here are some other ways to tell if you're struggling with emotional fatigue:

- Have you been feeling irritable, unable to cope, annoyed at every demand and intrusion? *If so, you're suffering from emotional fatigue.*
- Are there things you need to do in your life that you're not doing? I'm not talking about procrastination—we all have long lists of things that we haven't gotten around to doing. *But if you're not doing things that you really need to do, then you're suffering from emotional fatigue.*
- Do you feel that with your life in general (not just in one particular part of your life) you're just going through the motions, phoning it in, pushing yourself to do what has to be done even though your heart isn't in it? *If so, you're suffering from emotional fatigue.*
- Has it been more than a week since you did something for yourself that took some effort but gave you real enjoyment? I'm talking about making an effort, not just watching TV or talking on the phone. And I'm talking about real enjoyment, not about a meaningless moment of pleasure. *If it's been more than a week, you're suffering from emotional fatigue.*

If you're emotionally fatigued, I have some important news for you. In all the years I spent researching energy, my most significant finding is that the amount of emotional energy that you have is under your control. It's not about your upbringing. It's not about your genetic makeup. It's not about your personality. You can increase your emotional energy whenever you want. All the potential emotional energy in the world already exists inside you. It's all about how you approach life. You just have to do what people who are filled with emotional energy do. But you shouldn't delay—waiting will only make things worse.

And you should also know that you have lots of company.

Welcome to the Club

It's important for you to know that, based on data from the National Institutes of Health, one out of eight adults is in the same low-energy state you're in. This makes sense. After all, the number-one question people bring to their family doctor is "Why do I feel so blah?"

We don't realize there are so many fatigued people because of a kind of optical illusion. We compare how drained we feel inside with how energetic other people seem to be. *Seem*. But are they really? Don't be so sure. Most people keep their exhaustion hidden.

I learned an important lesson about the danger of comparing your insides to other people's outsides when I was seventeen. I was studying acting in Manhattan that summer with the great Herbert Berghof. He was one of the premier acting teachers, on a par with Lee Strasberg and Stella Adler. Naturally I had a crush on this handsome, dynamic older man. Somehow we fell into a routine of my driving him home after class.

That day he'd been lecturing on the need to maintain an intense connection with your audience. I asked, "How do you get that kind of energy night after night?" He sighed. It was late on a dark, warm, soft New York evening. We were parked in front of his house on Washington Square. The top of my convertible was down. Something made him let down his guard.

"I'll tell you the truth," he said. "I only feel really alive for maybe five minutes a day. Those are golden moments, and I never know when they're going to come. The rest of the time . . ." He sighed again. "That's why they call it acting. Conveying the illusion of an energy you know about only because of how much you wish you had it."

I've heard of faking orgasms. He'd been faking energy!

My years as a researcher and clinician have taught me that my wonderful teacher was not the only person to spend his days looking for energy and pretending he's got it. Coffee merchants and motivational speakers would go out of business tomorrow if we all had as much energy as we pretend we do. The screen world is filled with images of people bursting with energy. The real world is filled with real people desperately seeking more energy. That's what you and I are. We are energy seekers.

You'd be surprised at how many of the things we do are actually expressions of our search for energy. These go way beyond our search for more energy from physical sources. They include our seeking new experiences, our passion for authenticity, our attempts to connect with others, our need for change, our love of fun, our hunger for travel, and our restless creativity. All of these mark us as energy seekers.

But others have found what you're seeking, and you can find it too.

How You Can Get More Emotional Energy

What, then, is the secret of high-energy people? They live in the same world you and I do. But high-energy people consistently focus on increasing their emotional energy. That's their secret.

Many of us make a mistake: We say that to have emotional energy, you have to have a positive attitude. Well, yes, people with emotional energy do have a positive attitude. But you can't just tell yourself to have a positive attitude. We've all tried that, and it doesn't work. That's because emotional energy comes from the things you do to give yourself emotional energy.

So much of life is like this, isn't it? People do well in an area they care about—losing weight, making money, taking fabulous vacations—because they make it a priority and follow certain guidelines. Everyone who does the things that give emotional energy *gets* emotional energy.

This book contains everything that works to increase your emotional energy. After years of research, I've discovered that there are twenty-five simple, specific, effective shortcuts to boost your emotional energy. These are the secrets of high-energy people. Ideally, you'd have all of them working for you. But you certainly need as many as you can get. Your body has certain nutritional requirements. The twenty-five secrets are the requirements for emotional energy.

You *particularly* need whatever emotional energy boosters are missing in your life. To help you with this, with each emotional energy booster I've included a diagnostic question that will help you see whether that one is needed by you right now.

The energy boosters come in a certain order: Those that come first give the most energy most easily to the most people. This makes sense. If you're emotionally exhausted, you want quick results with a minimum of effort. But this isn't a step-by-step program. We're all unique. What you need, what will work best for you, will be different than for anyone else.

Here's how to use this book. Use whichever energy boosters feel right to you now. Trust yourself. At other times others will feel right. The secrets that work best for you are the ones you like to do the most and the ones that are easiest for you. I wish we could say that the foods that tasted best were best for us. But the fact that an emotional energy booster appeals to you is a guarantee that it will help you.

You Can Get the Emotional Energy You Need

Everything that gives you energy is good and needs to be embraced. Everything that saps it is bad and needs to be avoided. When you're not taking care of your emotional energy, you're not taking care of your life.

So, okay. No more neglecting your emotional energy. You don't need to. You're now holding in your hands everything you need to get more.

What I love most about life is how full it is of wonderful things, like a huge, varied, beautiful garden. There are wonderful people, wonderful things to do, wonderful discoveries to make. The worst thing about life is that often this garden seems to lie out of reach behind a heavy locked door. Maybe others have access to all the wonderful things, but you don't feel you do.

Emotional energy is the key that unlocks the door to that garden. So whether you're in a temporary slump or you've always thought of yourself as needing more energy, you will experience yourself as a high-energy person as you discover the secrets of emotional energy.

1

The Hell with Other People's Expectations

Emotional Energy Booster #1

What's an ideal energy source? One that's cheap and powerful. One that's easy to get but gives you a lot. One that works fast.

That's what this secret of emotional energy is. Talk about shortcuts! All you'll have to do here is flick a mental switch, and you've immediately eliminated an energy drain and at the same time tapped into a powerful energy source.

And interestingly enough, this is one of the most frequent ways high-energy people give themselves a big hit of emotional energy. You'll rarely find someone with high emotional energy who isn't using this secret.

Too Much to Live Up To

Most of the people who are important to us have very specific expectations that they want us to live up to. Not only do parents want their kids to be successful, but they often want their kids to live a certain way or have a certain kind of career. People want their spouses to be ambitious or nurturing or social. People want friends to be cool or funny or endlessly helpful.

When the expectations people have of you are the same as your own, then your life can feel in harmony. But when the people who are important to you have expectations that are out of sync with what you want and what you need for yourself, then you could be going through life with a terribly draining burden on your emotional energy.

Here are three people who found a wonderful increase in their emotional energy. But first they had to confront the burden of other people's expectations that they were carrying around.

Sandi, 26: "Lots of us have parents who put really high expectations on us. My mother was a model. I can tell you it can really be hard to be the daughter of a model. Maybe we should form a support group—recovering daughters of models. The point is, she was beautiful, and still is. Which is great for her. But I had to be beautiful too. As her looks faded, I was supposed to give her glory because of my looks. But a couple of the wrong genes got into me. In real life I'm okay-looking, but in the pages of a fashion magazine I'd look like a warthog. The thing is that every day as I got ready to leave the house, at some point I'd look in the mirror and I'd see that I'm not spectacularly beautiful and I'd get this feeling like when you get really bad news. I'd drag that bad feeling around with me all day."

Joseph, 32: "It was like they were telling me I'd be a murderer if I did what I wanted to do. My grandfather started our textile importing business. My father built it up. And so of course I'd carry on. Because if I didn't, who would? And if I didn't, it would be like I'm murdering my father and grandfather. Maybe if I'd wanted to be a doctor they could've accepted what I wanted for my life, but I studied special ed. The thought that I'd kill our family's dreams to be someone who works with emotionally disturbed kids just seemed weird. So I went to work at the family business every day. I made business trips. I learned about buying silk. But I felt like I was feeding the family business with my lifeblood. I felt drained."

Lisa, 43: "It seems like everyone I care about has expectations for me. My mom's a housewife and she felt she missed out on something, so she drilled into me that I had to have a career. And my dad thought I was smart, so he wanted me to have a big-deal kind of career. Well, I'm a teacher, and that's not good enough for them. They make these comments like when am I going to get my Ph.D., like I'm supposed to be on track for becoming a principal. My in-laws, God bless them, have this Martha Stewart view of life where I'm supposed to entertain and make a beautiful home. I know my husband wants that too. But he also likes the money I make. And I think he's a little afraid of being married to someone who's 'just a housewife.' No matter what I did I couldn't win. The pressure was exhausting—I was always looking into their faces and feeling their judgments."

There you have it. Three people struggling with emotional exhaustion. Why? Joseph and Lisa burned enormous amounts of energy trying to be who their families wanted them to be. Sandi knew she couldn't be what her mother wanted, but she lived with daily disappointment in herself because she'd bought into her mother's expectations.

Why is this so exhausting? Suppose you had a job, and you and a coworker did the same tasks. But by some bizarre twist 80 percent of your paycheck kept ending up in his pocket. You're both working hard, but he gets most of the benefit of your work. How long could you go on that way?

That's what happens when you try to live your life according to someone else's expectations. You're supposed to get satisfaction from the way you live your life. Maybe not every minute, but in general you have a right to expect satisfaction from life. But when someone else's expectations determine how you live, it's the other person, not you, who gets the emotional satisfaction from your efforts. You're putting out energy, but you're starving to death emotionally.

Diagnostic Question #1

Do you often feel angry with someone important to you because that person tells you how you should live your life? Do you feel that people are disappointed in you? Do you live in fear of other people's judgments of you?

*A **yes** answer to any of these questions means that this secret will give you a big boost of emotional energy.*

You Made the Jail, and You Hold the Key

What keeps you and me stuck with this—and most of us are stuck here to some degree—actually has nothing to do with other people. Everyone in the world has expectations for everyone else. So what? The problem is that we've somehow *bought into* other people's expectations for us.

This is the important point. Yes, Sandi, Joseph, and Lisa saw very clearly that someone else's expectations were putting pressure on them. No denial there. Where the problem arose was *in the extent to which they agreed with those expectations*. Sandi spent years thinking "Yes, of course I should be beautiful. I can see why my mother would be so disappointed. I'm disappointed too." But was Sandi really disappointed in herself? Was that really what Sandi expected of herself?

Joseph too spent years agreeing with his family's beliefs. Yes, if he left the family business, it might fail, and that would be a very bad thing and make him a very bad person.

Lisa, in spite of how much she resented that pressure, basically agreed that a woman should have a fabulous career and be a fabulous home-maker all at the same time. She directed her disappointment at herself for not living up to this.

And this is how Sandi, Joseph, Lisa, and so many of us give ourselves burdens that exhaust us. We can't bring ourselves to say no. We can't draw a line between ourselves and the people we care about.

So here's how to plug a big leak fast and get a big surge of energy:

Emotional energy booster #1
Stop buying into someone else's expectations for you.

You don't have to do this with everyone in your life. Just start with one person whom you feel has laid a heavy weight of expectations on you for who you should be or how you should be.

Then say something like this to *yourself:* "I understand what this person expects. But I don't expect that for myself. I'm sorry if he or she is disappointed, but I have to make sure my top priority is that I live up to my own expectations." This is a personal declaration of independence. It's for you to know. And that's all. You don't have to go to that person and have a confrontation. You don't ever have to tell them. But you do need to declare to yourself that from now on what counts is living up to your own expectations. Other people's expectations are not such a big deal to you anymore.

And you have to really mean it.

What you'll see is how much the way you lived your life was permeated by this person's expectations for you. You'll discover how much your guilt or your sense of duty or your fear of doing things for yourself kept you stuck trying to live up to the other person's expectations.

We rarely live in a prison that we haven't made ourselves. But it's the prison you've made yourself that you can break out of most easily. If you're the one holding you there, nothing prevents you from getting out.

The Gift of Freedom

What's the worst that can happen if you stop buying into someone else's expectations for you? Someone who's not you will be disappointed. But *you* will feel wonderful. Your sense of relief will be immediate and enormous. It will fill you full of emotional energy.

Sandi did this. All it took was a flash of insight. One day, after she and her husband had made love, he said she was beautiful. He'd said stuff like that before, of course. Sandi had always put it down to his wanting to get back in her pants. But this day the nuttiness of what she'd been doing to herself suddenly came clear. "Why should I be disappointed in the way I look when the man I love likes the way I look? Why do I need to have expectations for myself that stab me in the heart every time I look in the mirror when I can look in his eyes and feel his love?"

And Sandi let go of the expectation that she needed to be beautiful the way her mother wanted her to be. She couldn't change her mother. But she changed herself. It felt as though a hundred-pound weight had been taken off her shoulders. In the weeks after, her friends kept commenting on how good Sandi was looking. Of course. Emotional energy is the ultimate beauty secret.

Lisa was surrounded by many people's expectations. They crowded around her like flies at a picnic. Then one day Lisa was talking to her third-grade class about what they wanted to be when they grew up. The room filled up with images of firemen, ballerinas, astronauts, and veterinarians. And some wanted to be teachers. For the kids these were all aspirational images of hope and freedom. Lisa thought, "I'm a teacher, but I'm disappointed in myself. So should I tell these kids to forget about teaching?"

And then it hit her. Lisa wanted to be exactly what she was. She liked her life. She liked herself. She had everything she needed to be happy. Being a teacher was something to be proud of. She didn't want to be more than a teacher. She didn't want to be more than a slapdash homemaker. And so she decided to let go of all the expectations from other people that had invaded her. The next time she threw together a dinner she was able to say to herself, "They want me to make a gourmet feast. But I'm happy with the lasagna recipe from the back of the box."

Part of her stopped trying so hard. Part of her let go of her disappointment in herself for not trying harder. She just let herself be herself. And for the first time in years Lisa felt a surge of energy that allowed her to begin thinking about doing fun things for herself. She started enjoying life.

Joseph was in the toughest trap. It seemed to be all or nothing: totally commit to the family business or leave it completely. Everyone in his life expected him to sacrifice himself on the altar of the family business. And Joseph believed that if he walked out, the business might collapse.

But no one is ever completely trapped. Joseph made the tiniest mental shift, and that's the key for everyone. He basically gave himself permission not to buy into their expectations. "They want me to want this, and I've been beating myself up for not wanting it. But I didn't want it and that doesn't make me a bad person. I'm not going to walk out immediately. Not now. Too many people would get hurt. But I can let go of my sense that I *should* be wanting this for me. I don't, and that's all there is to it. And in fact there are plenty of people of my generation in my family who can run this business and who'd love the chance. I can start grooming them for it immediately. Then one day soon, when the time is right, I can walk away."

That was all he did. Instead of beating himself up, he accepted himself for not wanting to dedicate his life to the family business. But deep down, he freed himself from a terrible sense of disappointment and conflict. He wasn't a failure for wanting to work with emotionally disturbed kids. He was himself. That slight shift released a weight from Joseph's heart, and he felt lighter than he had in years.

Setting Yourself Free

You are probably burdened by a specific expectation from a specific person. Your mother or father, or your spouse or lover—these people have lots of expectations for you.

So, who is one person in your life right now whose expectations are a problem for you? Who in your life makes you feel just a little more emotionally exhausted because of your sense of their disappointment in you?

Now try to state the other person's expectation for you in one simple sentence. For example, "My partner expects me to be slim and trim." Or "My dad wants me to have what he calls a 'real career.'"

Next try to identify how you yourself have signed on to the same expectation. It's not that you *really* want this for yourself. It's just that you've gone along with something that you don't truly believe is you. For example, you've worked hard to lose weight the way your partner wants, but when you're honest with yourself you can see that you feel resentful, deprived, and inauthentic. Or perhaps you've agreed with your dad that you should want a "real career," but deep down you don't believe it, at least not for yourself.

This is the most important step—seeing how you've signed on to someone else's expectation that in your heart you don't agree with. Once you can see this, you're free. Then what you do is say *to yourself,* "That's fine for them, but that's not me. *I no longer have to expect this of myself.*"

Who's the boss of you? You're the boss of you. No big fight. No wrenching life changes. All you're doing is acknowledging to yourself what you really feel and believe, and yet this has the power to free up enormous amounts of your emotional energy.

2

Giving Yourself a Life
Filled with Meaning

Emotional Energy Booster #2

Very, very few people stagger around hollow-eyed saying in a tragic tone of voice, "My life has no meaning." Most of us, even most people who are feeling emotionally fatigued, can point to things that give their life meaning. So, yes, we do have meaning in our lives.

But at the same time a surprising number of us do have a *problem* with meaning in our lives. Yes, there's a foundation of meaning, often from wanting to take care of our families. Yet we don't *feel* the sense of having a life charged with meaning, not the way we used to, not the way we'd like to. It's not a complete lack of a sense of meaning—it's just a shortage. But that shortage is enough to have a terrible effect on our emotional energy.

Without meaning, there's no real reason or reward for what you do. And if you do something for no reason and with no hope of reward, how in the world is that supposed to energize you?

So it's important that you pause and think about the next question for a moment. Be honest. You'll be glad you did.

> ### *Diagnostic Question #2*
>
> *Did you have a sense of meaning at some point in your life that you no longer have to the same degree? Is there a staleness or an emptiness in your life now that bothers you?*
>
> *A **yes** answer to either of these questions means that this secret will give you a big boost of emotional energy.*

I'm going to tell you about some people who thought they'd lost a sense of meaning. But don't worry. Their stories have happy endings. If you can see what they saw, your story will also have a happy ending.

The Meaning of Your Life Cannot Be Taken for Granted

We make a huge mistake about how this whole meaning business works. We think meaning just happens. We think that the meaning of life is a given. Imagine our surprise when it goes away!

A sense of meaning is never handed to any of us on a silver platter. You can never count on your sense of purpose always being there for you without any effort on your part, no matter how rich and deep that sense of purpose is, no matter how committed you are to it.

Let me tell you about a rabbi I knew when I was a kid. He was a saintly man. As wise and learned as he was, even more he was a good man, kind and gentle and sweet. Everyone who knew him loved him. He lived in my building. And what happened to him stayed with me my whole life.

He was in his sixties then. The Holocaust had been over for about ten years. I guess the rabbi had thought long and deep and studied and prayed endlessly all those years about what it meant that millions of Jews and millions of other people had been killed so easily, wiped away the way a puff of breath blows away dust from a tabletop.

And one day he simply stopped believing. God had been for him a fact as real and solid as a house, and one day God vanished for this rabbi. He suddenly felt he'd dedicated his life to nothing. There simply could not be a God, he concluded, who let such a thing happen.

He'd counted on meaning always being there for him. He'd never counted on having to find meaning for himself. He continued to dress like an ultra-Orthodox Jew, out of respect and habit. But prayers and synagogue and observance of rituals all ended. He was still kind to everyone, but instead of having a congregation the only flock he tended were the pigeons who came for his crumbs in the park where I talked to him every day.

But we can never take our sense of meaning for granted. Otherwise our energy is in peril. And when our energy is in peril, we are in peril.

You're in Charge of the Meaning of Your Life

The meaning of your life is like being in shape. You have to make it happen. You have to renew it, revive it, refocus it. Yet we don't. We can't imagine how. But there are ways. And I'll show you what they are soon.

Sometimes what happens to people is less dramatic than what happened to the rabbi. But lots of us find meaning and then something terrible happens and we lose it, like when you built a tower of blocks as a kid and you were so proud, but before you could show it to your mother it collapsed.

That's what happened to Michelle. She looks fine, like the strong, sensitive person she is. But she's been drifting, and it feels as though her emotional energy is gone.

Michelle, 28: "The whole time I was growing up my life was music. I was going to be a classical violinist. There's a whole generation of exciting young women violinists who inspired me. I practiced for hours a day just so I could play beautifully. This might sound corny, but I wanted a chance to give voice to all the beautiful music there is in the world.

"And I was making it too. I had a scholarship to Juilliard, and when I graduated I had a lot of offers and opportunities.

"I guess it was over a period of a year that I realized I was getting arthritis. Which is ridiculous for a person my age. I couldn't believe it was happening. So you tell yourself you just need to practice more. But that's not it. What's happened is that the bottom has fallen out of your life.

"I looked at my violin, and it was useless to me. I wasn't sitting around feeling sorry for myself. I moved on. I taught music, and there's a lot of satisfaction in that. But I just didn't feel that my life had meaning the way it used to. I drifted through my days. I felt empty. What can I say?"

In one way meaning is like love. It's terrible to lose it, as the rabbi and Michelle did. It's perhaps worse never to have experienced it, like Jack.

If you'd wanted to find Jack most days, the best place to look would have been on the golf course. It sounds like a good life. But Jack carried around a deep yet visible sense of discontent.

Jack, 56: "I worked hard all my life to make a lot of money, and I did. Most of my early years on Wall Street were . . . I wouldn't say they were a lot of fun, but they were fueled by a sense of challenge and competitiveness. I'm one of those guys who said that whoever has the most toys at the end wins.

"The game was interesting, and it was nice to have a lot of money. But I guess my mistake was thinking it would add up to something. I took it for granted that when I got to the end of the rainbow I'd feel a sense of meaning from it all. But it felt very empty.

"I know most people envy what I have—and don't get me wrong, I'm grateful as hell for it—but it doesn't amount to anything beyond money. You want to know how it felt to be me? I felt again like the lost kid I was when I was twenty-two and didn't know what I wanted to do with my life. And when you feel lost like that, you feel tired, you feel restless, nothing really matters to you, and all the money in the world can't make it better. Even golf was a lot more fun when it was a special treat. But when it was all I did, it became like going to work, except that it wasn't a job I'm good at."

I know no one's feeling sorry for Jack. He's made his bed, and now he has to lie in it, except that it's a gold-plated, mink-lined bed. Poor baby.

But if you look past the money, you see a situation lots of us can relate to. I included Jack almost to challenge your sense of empathy. And why not empathize? You'd feel bad too if you thought you'd find meaning in something, and you worked hard, and in the end it felt empty of meaning.

When it comes to the story of emotional energy in his life, Jack is like the woman who worked hard to bring up her family as best she could, and then the kids grew up and left home, and instead of a harvest of meaning, she's harvesting only a sense of emptiness. Jack is like the guy who works in a social service agency all his life to help the disadvantaged, and he's proud of what he's done, but after many years his community is still filled with disadvantaged people and he feels that instead of having built an ark, all he's done is bail out a leaky boat.

It's not depression. It's not burnout. Instead it's an honest, heartfelt assessment of what years of work and effort feel like they add up to. Did you ever go on vacation to somewhere special and spend a lot of money, yet it turned out to be actually a rather disappointing vacation? That's happened to many of us. Well, let's be honest. That's what happens to our sense of meaning. We hoped we'd find it, maybe we thought we had it, and instead we're disappointed in what we really got.

If this is true for you, you'd better not pretend it isn't. Only accepting it will make it possible for you to get more emotional energy.

How to Give Your Life Meaning

Watching people struggle to find meaning in their lives, I found that there are many solutions that work. One of them will be right for you. For example, when's the last time you asked yourself, "What is something I could do, or do differently, that would give me more meaning in my life?" This basic question is an excellent way to begin. All you have to do is answer as best you can and then do your best to carry out your answer. You don't need to come up with a brilliant answer. Just by asking it, you reorient your entire being in such a way that you immediately get more emotional energy.

Another thing you can do is to assume you've lost your sense of meaning for no reason other than you've gotten lazy and distracted. You know very well what's given your life meaning in the past. You just have to renew your connection to that now. Maybe you've lived to take care of your family, for example. But the kids got older and your spouse became more independent. And you got busy with other things. But who's to say that you're not as important to your family as you were before, if not more so? Reach out to the people in your family. Make some nice things happen. Just go out there and recapture the sense of meaning you used to have.

Another straightforward solution to the issue of meaning is to think about what you care about and then do something about it. That's all meaning is: caring plus a network of actions that ties your life to what you care about. No matter what it is, no matter how tiny or insignificant it may seem to others, if your caring is real and if you do things to bring your caring into the fabric of your everyday life, you will feel a sense of meaning return.

What about the rabbi, Michelle, and Jack? What solutions did they develop? Their roads were hard, yet they came up with great solutions.

One is to turn loss into gain. A classic example of this is the women who founded Mothers Against Drunk Driving (MADD). A beloved child was taken away in a senseless accident. Anyone who's been in this situation feels that the meaning in her life has been lost. But instead of suffering helplessly, these women plucked a rose of meaning from the midst of cruel thorns of loss. Where their children had died, they would work to save the lives of other mothers' children.

Jack did something very similar, turning something that took energy from him into something that gave him energy. He thought about the empty gilded cage he was rattling around in, and he thought about all the young men and women on Wall Street happily but unknowingly building such cages for themselves. And he decided to work to help them. Maybe they weren't the neediest people in the world. But they were *his* people. And feeling empty is feeling empty no matter who you are.

With a couple of equally rich friends living lives equally drained of meaning, Jack started reaching out to Wall Street guys and gals to show them how to donate time and money to underprivileged young people who were having trouble starting their lives. Below the surface Jack's goal was to help his friends by helping them find a way to discover projects they cared about that weren't just about making money.

Jack made that a major part of his effort—educating money-driven men and women about the need to find meaning by helping others.

Now Jack's emotional energy is sky high.

Anyone can do this. It doesn't have to be on Jack's scale. It doesn't have to take much money. *Identify what you've had taken away from you. Then help someone else find something like that. That's the basic principle.* Jack thought he'd been building something that would last. Now he's helping others build something that really does have a chance to last.

You can't redeem the past. But you can redeem the future.

Michelle might've done something like this, maybe working with disabled musicians or children. Instead, she found a different solution: continuing the struggle regardless of the payoff. You were working hard, and life made a monkey of you? Okay. Then you carry on as a monkey. You find meaning from carrying on in spite of the fact that it seems as though you've lost meaning. You get meaning from enduring, from persisting, from keeping up the struggle no matter what, and if one path is blocked, you find another. No one can take your meaning from you because you're not a quitter.

For Michelle this meant continuing to make music. Of course she could no longer use her hands to play. But you don't need much dexterity to write music for others to play. It wasn't easy. She was no Mozart. From being a gifted performer she went to being a composer of no proven talent.

"But," Michelle said, "so what? I'd thought it was about winning, but it's really about playing the game, staying in the game, finding a way to hang on no matter what." You have to let go of your need to win, or at least win a specific prize. Instead you embrace the struggle.

Again, anyone can do this. *The principle here is that when your house gets blown down, you build it up again, and if it keeps getting blown down, you keep building it up. You have meaning as long as you keep struggling.* No one can take your meaning away from you unless you take your own willingness to struggle away from yourself.

What this means for you is that you keep going anyway even though you think something has destroyed your sense of meaning, and you find your meaning in keeping going. You're the person no one can stop, and if something does stop you, you just find another way.

The rabbi could've done this. Yes, he'd lost his sense of meaning. But who said he had to stop being a practicing rabbi? He could've said, "God no longer makes sense to me, but that makes my faith all the more special." His congregation would've still loved him.

But the rabbi found still another solution. Again, the right solution is the one that works for you. What worked for him was to discover that you can find meaning by living without meaning. The meaning of your life comes from simply living your life.

It sounds like a paradox, but it really isn't. You can enjoy life without any sense of meaning beyond simply enjoying life. You enjoy the moment. You enjoy what you find pleasure in. At the end of Voltaire's *Candide,* after a series of harrowing losses, Candide famously decides to cultivate his garden. Who knows what anything means, perhaps? Who knows if you can ever find the ultimate meaning? But you can grow a rose and enjoy its perfect shape and color. You can grow a tomato and enjoy its ripe, juicy flavor. And at the end of all of this, what was the meaning of your life? The meaning of your life was that you received the gift of life and enjoyed it. Nothing more. But nothing less.

When I was a child this rabbi was a figure of mystery, not just to me but to everyone in my neighborhood—a rabbi who stopped being a rabbi but in some sense was still a rabbi. He sat in the park with the pigeons, and I saw that he talked to the children and they trusted him and the normally suspicious mothers in the neighborhood seemed to trust their children with him.

So I went one day and stood near the rabbi, shy, not my usual talkative self. I remember the rabbi said to me, "It's a beautiful day, don't you think?" He asked it like a real question, as though he really wanted me to think about how beautiful the day was. No one had ever talked to me about a beautiful day before. What a revelation. There were days that were beautiful! I solemnly agreed with him. Then he asked me, "Don't you think the pigeons would like it if we fed them?" Another revelation. I'd seen people feeding the pigeons before, but this was a new idea. The pigeons like it when you feed them. You can make the pigeons happy. Wow!

So we tossed bread crumbs, and for the first time in my life I saw happy pigeons, where before I'd only seen pigeons. And all this was happening on a beautiful day, where before I'd only seen days.

Soon I had to go. I told the rabbi my mother was waiting for me. The rabbi thanked me for spending some time with him. He told me he'd enjoyed my being with him. Another new idea. We were refugees. I'd thought I was just a chore. But someone enjoyed me. There were beautiful days. Happy pigeons. And I could make people happy.

I walked home feeling without words that the world was suddenly a richer, more wonderful place filled with many happy things if you just cocked your head and looked at them with fresh eyes.

The rabbi understood that if the meaning of life is to enjoy life, it's even better if you enjoy it with someone else.

If this solution is right for you, you only need to let yourself do it. It can be hard to find meaning. So why exhaust yourself trying to find meaning in your life when you find enormous energy by stopping the search?

There's a wonderful scene in Woody Allen's *Manhattan* in which his character makes a long list of things that for him make life worth living.

Do that for yourself. What are all the things that could fill your life, all the pleasurable, satisfying things to do and experience?

That's your answer. The meaning that comes from enjoying your life.

Emotional energy booster #2
Take responsibility for finding meaning in your life.

If you wait for the universe to give you a sense of meaning, you'll be frustrated, and it will spoil your relationship with life and with yourself. But if you take responsibility for finding a sense of meaning, or even finding a way to live without it, that's your way of seeing that the universe is a place of abundance, where you can find meaning if you're willing to look for it.

Special Issue:

How Emotional Energy Works

Would you like to see actual raw emotional energy? Just follow a child around for a day. That child's happiness, intensity, resilience, playfulness, and curiosity are signs of high emotional energy. Parents and teachers marvel at children's energy, but physically children are actually weak and easily tired. It's their emotional energy that makes it possible for them to run almost any adult ragged and to bounce back from almost any difficulty.

Think about when you were most filled with a kind of happy, hopeful, creative, playful energy, when you had a lot to give and a tremendous capacity to receive. It was probably in your childhood.

That's how we all start life: as high-energy people, exuberant, *effervescent*. So why don't we stay that way? Bodies age, but the heart and mind and spirit don't. There's something wrong. We should all have the emotional energy of a happy child, and yet we don't. *What happens to us?*

There's an important clue for us in the following personal account.

Patti, 31: "I guess you could say that I had a disadvantaged background. My mother was a waitress and God knows she did her best, but she was on her own with me and my two brothers. By the time she got finished earning money to put a roof over our heads, she didn't have much left to give. We grew up in the projects. I didn't see a lot of hope there. I didn't see role models. Nobody in my little world expected much from me. I guess the big lesson I was taught was to be a good girl and do what you're told. No one saw me. No one knew me. I know my mother cared about me, but only as an organism, not as someone special. And that was a pretty discouraging message. No one was interested in me for who I was.

"So what happened? Thank God we lived three blocks from the public library. I don't remember when I first discovered it—maybe when I was around nine or ten—but it was like discovering a whole other world. In fact, almost every book I read pointed to a new world.

"It was about all the possibilities in life. It didn't matter what I read. Picture books. Storybooks. Later on, novels. Still later, nonfiction. Everyone I read about was having adventures and moving out from some small world to a larger, brighter, more interesting world. The people I read about were stuck in so many different ways, and yet they all found a way to get unstuck. Most of all—and I don't know how I picked up on this at such an early age—everyone I read about found a way to discover his own little dream. That's what the books were about. Discovering yourself, your dreams, running into obstacles, and then finding a way to make your dreams happen. And then you felt there was a place for you in the world.

"Those books saved my life. It's not just that they were big arrows pointing to a wonderful world out there. It's more that they were arrows pointing to something in me that was special and wonderful and that would have a place in the big world out there. I never lost that message of hope."

The Battle for Emotional Energy

Patti found a way to save herself. Everyone finds a different way. But what do all these different ways have in common?

All of us want to feel at home in the world, safe and hopeful, happy and comfortable. We want to feel we're living in a world that fits us. What emotionally exhausts us is the struggle to be ourselves in a world that has its own, very different ideas about who we are and what we're supposed to do.

Your emotional energy system is very different from your physical energy system. From the point of view of physical energy, you're just a machine. You need fuel, the best fuel possible. You need to be well maintained. When you eat well, sleep well, and get enough exercise, that's just what you're doing.

Your emotional energy system works completely differently. It's really *you,* and you're not a machine at all. You're a *self,* a special, creative, dynamic, happy, hopeful, wonderful self. You are, deep down and in your essence, the perfect, unique person God created. But why did God create you specifically? To make special use of this world and to enjoy it to your fullest. You're not a drone, a tool, a means to an end, or an animal just like the others in the herd. You are *you,* and there's no one else like you. As you'll see in a moment, this has enormous implications for your emotional energy.

Compare what happens to our physical energy with what happens to our emotional energy as we grow up. For the average adult, physical energy reaches a peak in early adulthood and then very slowly diminishes.

It's a different story when it comes to emotional energy. Compare the inner energy of a child with the inner energy of the typical adult in his thirties. In most cases, the loss of emotional energy is large and striking. Even though the adult has some emotional energy, there's been a major dulling of energy compared to when he was a kid. More cynicism, more wariness, less passion, diminished ability to have fun, loss of trust, loss of self-confidence.

Quick take: a bunch of kids sitting around eating lunch together. What are the kids talking about? Probably nonsense, but they're having a ton of fun. Now consider a bunch of adults sitting around eating lunch together. What are the adults talking about? Too often they're complaining, talking about their problems. What a stark difference between the two groups.

What is it about leaving childhood that causes our emotional energy to diminish so much faster than our physical energy?

Since human beings first appeared on this planet, children have presented a challenge to society. High spirits are great, but adults need children to buckle down eventually. Life is hard, and it requires work and self-denial.

Think about the messages you got growing up. Few were "You're fine just the way you are." Most were "When are you going to straighten out and get with the program?"

A kid wants to do *what* he wants to do the *way* he wants to do it. But adults want kids to do what *they* want kids to do, and to do it the *right* way. So the transition from childhood to adulthood is marked by adults giving children the message that they're not okay the way they are. There's something wrong with what they want and with the ways they do things.

This is what you and I and every other kid has had to deal with. We accept the demands adults make on us growing up. But it has a terrible impact on our emotional energy to be constantly told that there's something wrong with us for being ourselves. Take the world of relationships, for example. A girl might start out relating to boys in whatever way feels right to her. But social pressure, the fears of her parents, and the way boys are discourage her from continuing to do things in a spontaneous way.

What's the emotional trajectory of someone who's been dating from fifteen to thirty? It's a transition from being herself to being some other way—a self constructed out of social pressure, the advice in women's magazines, dating "rules," and whatever lessons she's learned. From confidence to caution, from hope to cynicism, from spontaneity to calculation.

What happens to young women in relationships happens to everyone in every realm—more or less, but it happens. And it robs us of our energy. Your emotional energy doesn't care about how successful you are in worldly terms. *Your emotional energy only cares about how successful you are at being yourself.*

It takes a lot more energy *not* to do things your own way. You have to constantly monitor yourself: This is where the painful self-consciousness of adolescence comes in. You have to rein yourself in: This is where the tight, emotionally flat behavior of job applicants and people on first dates comes in. You have to try to do things in an uncomfortable, unfamiliar way.

Have you ever had a tennis coach or golf instructor try to get you to change your swing? If so, you know how painful and difficult it is. You know how hard you resist. You know how discouraged you get. You know how it sucks the fun out of the game. If you manage to change, maybe it was worth it. But whenever you try to turn something against its natural direction, it consumes an inordinate amount of energy, and too often the payback is limited.

You can see how life creates energy seekers. Unable to feel completely ourselves in the world, we're always struggling to find a way to feel more ourselves. We want to live more authentically, in a way that's more natural to who we really are. The question is, Will we find what we're looking for?

Of course we will. As depleted as we feel sometimes, one of the best things I know about life is that it's filled with opportunities for increasing our energy. You can always do something to get more. Every one of the energy boosters in this book works because it helps you be more yourself, more truly you. It makes the world feel more comfortable and natural to you. And the more you are yourself, the more emotional energy you have.

3

Prayers That Really Work

Emotional Energy Booster #3

They say there are no atheists in a foxhole. That's probably true. And everyone has found himself in some kind of foxhole at one time or another. You feel under the gun, threatened, doomed, scared, humiliated, weak. You don't know what to do. You don't know where to turn.

This is the kind of situation where your emotional energy sinks to a low ebb. Sure, you've worked hard, kept your hopes up, tried your best. But you're still in a state of weakness and fear. How the hell do you keep up your emotional energy in a situation like that? Most people turn to the ultimate energy source—God. They pray. But then what?

Diagnostic Question #3

When you pray, does it give you a measurable boost? And do you typically turn to prayer specifically to feel better, happier, more alive?

    A **no** *answer to either of these questions means that this secret will give you a big boost of emotional energy.*

Some Prayers Work Better than Others

Prayer works. That's a fact. I know—sometimes when you pray for rain you don't get it. I'm not going to get into the theology of whether God *literally* answers prayers or not. But it's an incontrovertible finding of objective research that prayer makes people feel better. It does in fact give you emotional energy. And emotional energy is very often the miracle ingredient that helps people keep going and doing their part in making their prayers come true. After all, giving up is not the path to answered prayers.

This is how you can find yourself in a wonderful positive cycle: Prayer gives you emotional energy, emotional energy helps you take action, your actions make good things happen in your life.

But there's another research finding that's more important and yet less well known. Certain kinds of prayer work far better than others. This is a stark and surprising truth. From the point of view of emotional energy, some of us pray correctly and some of us don't know how to pray well at all.

By the way—and this might surprise you—you don't need to believe in God to pray and to get the benefits of prayer. Don't pray to God if you don't want to. Pray to the universe itself. Pray to all the forces outside of your control. Pray to whatever higher power there may be.

I'm approaching this as a clinician and a researcher. I'm not a member of the clergy, nor am I a theologian. God does not call me up on the phone and tell me His secrets. As far as I'm aware, God doesn't single me out for any direct communication at all, at least not more than anyone else. I'm like you. I peer into the darkness and do my best to find the ultimate truths of life.

So when I tell you that I've learned how to pray well, I'm talking from the point of view of studying flesh-and-blood men and women who've uttered millions of heartfelt prayers, and sometimes felt much better and sometimes not so much better. And the reason for this difference, it turns out, lies in how exactly these people prayed.

Needing the Secret of Emotionally Energizing Prayer

Let's follow the stories of two very different people who found themselves stuck in a dark pit in their lives. And who found a way to get the emotional energy to climb out.

Carol, 42: "I'm one of those people who always knew what they wanted to be when they grew up. I wanted to be a botanist. I loved growing things, and I loved the idea of finding a way to grow special things. Of course, life isn't the way you think it'll be when you're a kid. But I came pretty close.

"For the past ten years—more, really—I was working on a project to genetically engineer a better apple tree. One that put out better fruit faster. One that grew in warmer, drier climates, like many places in Africa. In fact, my mantra as I was working was that apple trees in Africa would be a blessing for the continent. No one knew if that was possible, but that's what we were looking for.

"So we kept creating specimens, making modifications, checking out the results, and creating more specimens. But it wasn't like physics or chemistry, where you can store formulas on a computer disk and back it up so that it can't be destroyed. My life's work was the actual plants I'd created.

"So when some nut set fire to our lab and burned it down, my life's work was destroyed. It would take me a decade to re-create those specimens. But by then other people in this field would've left me far behind. I was like one of those writers who works ten years on a book and there's only one copy of the manuscript and he accidentally leaves it in a taxicab and he never sees it again.

"I was devastated. I'd always been religious—I think of botanists as people who work alongside God. So of course I prayed. I wanted God to tell me why this had happened to me. And I wanted God to give me a grant, a good idea, something, anything. I was basically praying to God to give me back what I'd lost. I wanted God to turn back the clock.

"But no matter what I did, I still felt lost in the darkness. When God didn't give me back my trees, my praying left me feeling alone and helpless."

Carol's prayers weren't working for her to build up her emotional energy. Something similar happened to Ben.

Ben, 29: "When I was a kid I remember they'd tell you that you could be whatever you wanted to be and that you could rise as far as your potential would take you. And I remember thinking, 'Hey, that's a good deal.' So I'd listen to people like Dylan and Livingston Taylor and I thought I could do that. That's what I wanted to do. Be a kind of singer/poet. I had a good voice. I looked good. Good guitar player. I had a quirky little romantic view into things. I could see myself as a guy with a following and a career.

"But, jeez, man, what does it take? I'd been at it for eight years. My whole adult life. I'd get a gig, then I wouldn't get gigs. I had a CD out and everyone who heard it liked it, but no one heard it. But I couldn't get to do another. All this time I'd been doing temporary work and it wasn't leading me anywhere. It got to the point where my dream was more painful than not.

"I prayed, of course. You've got to stay tight with the Big Dude. I wasn't asking for much. I was just praying for the big break. I remember my top prayer was 'Please let someone powerful fall in love with my work.' Maybe my prayers were answered, but they were answered with silence. I felt abandoned by God."

It's sad. Two good, smart people praying for help like a drowning man praying for something to grab on to, but they weren't getting the emotional boost they needed.

Active Prayer

Here's what Carol and Ben should have done instead, based on what I've learned high-energy people actually do. I call it *active prayer*, the secret of prayer that's effective for building emotional energy.

First, your prayer has to be a genuine dialogue with God.

Carol and Ben weren't doing that. They were praying like children—helpless, self-absorbed, looking for magic. They made demands. They talked at God, not with Him. They treated God like a cosmic complaint department. If prayers like that gave people energy, fine. But they don't. They leave you standing there in the rain waiting for an umbrella to materialize. And the umbrella never comes, not for most of us, not often enough.

So the first key to active prayer is to talk to God as if you were genuinely interested in establishing a dialogue. As if God were a super-wise, super-good friend. I understand: God's not our buddy. We're mere mortals. We can't approach God on His level. But God can approach us on our level. So why don't we *be* on our own level and talk to God like a person?

How do you do this? Share your thoughts and feelings with God. Ask questions, by all means. But don't just sit there if you don't get an answer. Talk about answers that make sense to you and ask God what He thinks about your answers.

My teacher Martin Buber, author of the classic *I and Thou,* taught me this at the end of his life: You always have the responsibility and the opportunity to create a genuine dialogue by being your true self, approaching the other as a true self, and assuming that real communication is possible. When you do this, you break down all the barriers.

One thing we know for sure: God is not a chatterbox. So when we talk to God we have a lot of work to do to hold up our end of the conversation. Okay. But it is a conversation. And people who get energy from talking to God are engaged in that ongoing conversation. You're not having a conversation with someone when you say, "Give me this," "Do this for me," "Tell me why this happened." You have a genuine conversation when you share your thoughts and feelings, when you ask sincere questions, when you open-mindedly explore different possibilities, when you probe for the truth.

So as you're having this dialogue, imagine what God might say in response to what you said. That's all you can do to hold up God's side of the conversation—imagine what He might say. And who's to say that *isn't* what He'd say?

Suppose a relationship of yours hasn't worked out. You're heartbroken. So maybe you say to God, "I loved him so much. Why wasn't that enough?" Then you listen. And maybe somehow, from somewhere, you hear the sentiment "Love is not enough."

Now respond to His response. Maybe you have another question. Maybe it stimulates a thought in you. But that's all you need to keep a genuine dialogue going. Say things that show a desire for real dialogue. Imagine how God would respond. Respond to that. And keep it going.

Maybe all your questions will never be answered. But that's not what you need to get a big hit of emotional energy from praying. What makes the difference is the sense of engaging in a dialogue, that somehow, in some way, on some level, God will speak with you. You're not alone.

Of course, when we talk to God we are also looking for help. Establishing a dialogue means that God can help us with His wisdom. But usually we want more than that. We want real resources. We want that umbrella to materialize when we're standing out in the rain. And that too is a place where people make a big mistake. When you ask God to give you things or make your life different, you're asking God to be a better God. No wonder that goes over like a lead balloon!

Instead, the second key to active prayer is to ask God to help you be a better you. That's the *only* thing you should ask God to give you, at least from the point of view of getting more emotional energy.

Let's say you're looking for a job and you're starting to feel desperate. Lots of people have been in this situation. If you pray for God to actually produce a great new job for you, that won't give you emotional energy. Every day that God fails to drop a job in your lap will be a day in which you're disappointed with what God is doing for you. Instead of healing your relationship with the universe, you're poisoning it.

What high-energy people pray for are the inner resources we all need to be able to produce the outcomes we'd like. You want that great new job? Pray for perseverance. Pray for ways to understand better how to make a human connection with interviewers. Pray for the self-confidence to present yourself in the best possible light.

Whatever you're wanting to happen in your life, pray to be a better person in the ways that will bring about that outcome. Do you wish you had a happier marriage? Then pray to God to help you be a kinder, warmer, more understanding person.

Are you afraid that someone you love might die? Then pray to God to help you be strong and wise and smart and loving. Whatever the specific ways are that would make you better at dealing with the fact that a loved one might die, that's what you pray for.

Don't neglect the first key. Don't make it so that you're asking God to give you something. Instead, establish a dialogue. Ask, for example, "Why has it been so hard for me to persevere?" Or "What do I need to do to become a kinder person?" Or "How can I get more self-confidence?"

It's emotionally very moving to sincerely pray to be a better person. And somehow that in itself heals your emotional exhaustion.

Emotional energy booster #3
When you pray, have a real dialogue with God
and talk to Him about the ways in which
you'd like to be a better person.

Why Active Prayer Works

I don't know why God works the way He does, but I do know why *we* work the way we do. Outcomes are out of our hands. The more likely they are to be the kind of special outcomes we pray for—success, health, love—the more likely they are to be hard-to-come-by outcomes. There's no point in praying that you'll find a penny, because pennies turn up everywhere. But what do you think will happen if you pray to find a thousand dollars? How often do you find that lying around? The more specific and the more special the outcome is that you're praying for, the less likely you are to get it. Why set yourself up for discouragement?

Everything changes in your energy when you pray for changes in yourself. Now you are a fifty-fifty partner in making those changes happen. God helps those who help themselves. The only way you can help yourself that means anything is to change yourself. And the changes we're looking for happen faster and more easily when you feel you're not alone.

That's why active prayer is a secret of high-energy people.

Some people like to have specific words written out in advance when they pray. That's why we have the Lord's Prayer, the Shema Yisrael, the Manikka Vasagar—every religion has special prayers.

From the point of view of emotional energy, here's an excellent example of active prayer. I've pulled this prayer together from prayer phrases people have told me gave them the most emotional energy.

Dear God, my Lord and Friend, give me the vision and insight to see what's true in this confusing life of mine.

And out of all the things that I come to see are true, give me the intelligence to see what's most important.

And when I see what's most important, give me the understanding to know what to do about it, the strength to act on it, and the patience to see my actions through.

And help me become someone who can accept what can't be changed.

And help me develop the capacity to see what's good in my life and in this world.

And make me a kinder person.

Give this prayer a chance. Everyone who prays it for several days in a row sees his energy rising. But it's even better to engage in a spontaneous dialogue with God using your own words and feelings to talk to Him about what you're dealing with and ways you'd like to become a better person.

Carol and Ben made this shift. Look at the difference it made.

Carol: "I don't know how it happened, but I got tired of praying to God as if He were Santa Claus who could give me back all the trees that had been lost in the fire. I felt I needed someone to talk to about my despair. And I desperately needed the strength to go on. So I prayed for strength, and I talked about my life the way I would to my best friend. You know how you can have a conversation with a close friend and you realize that for the past half hour you were doing all the talking? That's what I did with God.

"Praying for strength and intelligence and goodness paid off. I don't know how it worked. Maybe it had something to do with asking God to help me find the gifts He'd given me that were already inside me. Praying for strength made me focus on my strength, and that made me feel strong.

"I found a whole new energy to resume my research. I'd gotten into this field to help people and because the work challenged me. And I was able to reconnect to that."

Ben: "I have a theory about artists that a lot of us deep down don't think we have what it takes. If we're successful, we think we're frauds. If we're not successful, we don't think we deserve to be successful. That's why the music business can be so discouraging. You know you're good, but you're afraid you're not good enough.

"I guess I got tired of praying for success. So one day I said, 'God, help me find my own voice. And help me see what I need to do to connect to people through my music. Real artists connect. I just want to be a better, more honest me.'

"That's all I focused on. Finding my voice and what I had to say. Finding whatever gold there was buried inside the dark mine of my talent. And focusing on, well, listening to people, actually. Because if you connect successfully, it's not because of what you say, but because of what you've heard people say that you're responding to.

"I was praying to find myself, really. Whatever that meant or led to. There was something about focusing on the truth in myself and the world I was trying to connect to that created a breakthrough. It's just been some little things so far. But I've gotten the energy I was looking for, and it's paid off. I'm starting to get more gigs. If I do something, it leads to something else. The world didn't change. I changed. And I thank God for that."

4

"I Did It My Way"

Emotional Energy Booster #4

We can all be more ourselves regardless of our environment. If a judge and a monk can do it, you and I can definitely do it.

Wendy, 44: "All my life I wanted to be a judge. I remember as a kid watching courtroom dramas on TV. From *Perry Mason* to *L.A. Law*, it wasn't the attorneys that got me excited, it was the judge sitting up there running the whole show. 'This is my courtroom,' he or she would always say at one point. And that always thrilled me.

"I was appointed a municipal court judge at a fairly young age. I'd been so eager to do whatever was necessary to get where I wanted that by the time I got there it wasn't me who'd arrived. It was some stranger who was very clever at saying and doing all the right things.

"I was incredibly elated my first day on the bench, but after that my mood, my energy, just sank and sank. After two years I was in a very low state. I felt miserable. This was my dream job, and yet as a case would drone on in front of me I'd make doodles of desert islands with palm trees and a castaway in a polka-dot bikini lying on the beach. That castaway was me. All I wanted was a one-way ticket to as far away as possible."

Like most people suffering from low emotional energy, Wendy didn't know what the problem was. She just knew she felt crummy. It almost feels like you have a chronic low-grade infection, except that it's your heart and mind and soul that are infected.

But Wendy was lucky. She found a way to get back the emotional energy she'd lost. We can all do what she did, each in our own way.

Wendy: "It hit me at one point that I was going to have to quit being a judge. The robe didn't fit, you might say. And when I saw that I was headed out the door, I kind of slammed on the brakes. 'What am I doing? I'm going to give up my childhood dream because . . . *why* exactly am I quitting? Because it doesn't feel right? *Why* doesn't it feel right?'

"Yeah, I was bored and it felt empty, but *why?*

"The solution kind of exploded in my head. 'I'm going to do things the way *I* want.' I didn't even know what that meant at first. I just knew I felt such a surge of energy at the thought that I could be myself. Then it hit me—I was really free. I mean, you have to follow the law. But musicians have to follow the laws of music. Why did I have to go along with the idea that the law meant I was in a straitjacket in how I behaved? Just because something's customary doesn't mean it's right. And it doesn't mean it's the law.

"I decided to push everything to the limit. As long as I wasn't guilty of misconduct, I was free. So I went for it. It was mostly little things. But they meant I was being myself. I put up a poster of Janis Joplin in my chambers. I said to myself, 'If anyone doesn't like it, screw them. Janis makes me happy.' I'd talk to people in my courtroom the way I wanted to talk to them. Who said I had to act like a TV judge? I let it all hang out. And I stopped wearing the robe. There's no rule that says a judge has to wear a robe. Anything that doesn't fatally compromise the dignity of the courtroom is acceptable.

"I had so much fun with all of that. It had a big impact on my work. I started getting involved in a number of alternative-sentencing movements. I felt alive and committed and happy. I'm sure Janis would've thought I was pretty tame. But I felt free. And it saved my life."

There are two key points to learn from Wendy. Many of us are losing emotional energy because of ways we're not letting ourselves be ourselves. As the great actor and singer Paul Robeson said, "You can only be a somebody when you're yourself." Do you want to destroy someone's emotional energy? Make them keep on feeling like they're not themselves day after day.

> ### *Diagnostic Question #4*
>
> *Are you happy with how much* you *there is in your life?*
>   *A* **no** *answer to this question means that this secret will give you a big boost of emotional energy.*

Come Home to Yourself

Some people make a mistake. They think that being yourself has something to do with flaunting your little quirks. But that makes it seem small and annoying. It's a much deeper issue.

The important point is that there can't be such a big gulf between who you are and the life you lead that your life doesn't feel like it's yours. You know how incredibly uncomfortable most of us feel in the dentist's chair? We feel that way even if we have a wonderful dentist who never causes any pain. It's not about pain. It's about spending an hour in an alien world where you have no place. If you could mail your teeth in to get worked on, you would.

But when you personalize your life, when you make your life a place where you can be yourself, when you do things the way you want to do them, your life feels like your home. And that is a tremendous source of emotional energy.

It's important to believe that there can *always* be more you in your life. Imagine the most restrictive environment you can. Like being a monk, for example. Don't they all have to act alike, think alike? Look again. There are basic rules monks have to follow, but beyond that even most monks are freer to be themselves than you might have thought.

Brother Andrew, 34: "I'm a Franciscan monk. This is a religious order with a very definite discipline. You have to live a life of poverty. And I have to confess that, like a lot of young men, I found the religious discipline tough to deal with. It's not supposed to be easy. But I started having big questions about my calling when I started feeling inauthentic in my vocation. Yes, we're dedicating our lives to serve God and to serve people. But the fact is that, like Popeye, I am what I am. It may be a sad fact, but it's true. It's not about my having a big ego. It's just that I can't serve God as anyone else but me. And yet at first I was living in the safety of this order feeling I couldn't be me. That was very painful. But was it a pain I needed to put up with? Was it helping me serve God or was it getting in my way?

"I kept thinking that St. Francis was disappointed in me. That's what held me back and made me run away from being myself. One year we went on a retreat, all of us from our monastery. A retreat for monks. Pretty intense. I was talking to an older Franciscan, and he said something very simple and powerful. He said, 'You weren't called upon to be St. Francis. You were only called upon to be Brother Andrew. That's hard enough. You don't have to make it harder by trying to be someone you're not.'

"That was so liberating. God called upon me to be *me* in His service.

As me. That meant I really could dedicate my heart and soul to God. I wasn't an impostor in my vocation. It was real because I was being me.

"And since then I've tried to be more fully myself whenever possible so that I could have a more immediate and satisfying relationship with God. For example, I've been much more entrepreneurial in our work with inner-city kids. I'm finding I can really take an initiative in searching out new ways to reach kids and in thinking up new ways to help them. The ultimate freedom for me is the freedom to serve God better. And so by being more myself, I've actually been helping to further the goals of our order."

How to Do Things Your Way . . . Not That You Need Instructions

Think about how you do something. Brushing your teeth, for example. You probably do it your own way. The way you're used to doing it. By now it's so easy to do it that way that you don't even think about it.

Now suppose someone gave you rules for a completely different way of brushing your teeth. Maybe using a different hand. Or maybe using a different motion of the toothbrush. It would be harder for you. It would take more time and energy. Not just physical energy, but a kind of mental energy because you'd have to pay attention in a whole new way.

It's like that with everything. Your way is the easy way. The natural way. The way that fits you. It takes the least energy from you. Now suppose we're talking about doing something much more important than brushing your teeth. Something you really care about. When you do it your way, it not only takes the least energy from you, it also gives you the most energy. We get energy from being ourselves. We quite literally turn ourselves on.

And whenever and wherever you're not being yourself, you spend extra energy doing it some other person's way and you starve yourself from getting emotional energy because the way you're doing it is alien to you.

We've all heard of soul-destroying jobs. Now you know why and how they destroy your soul. They don't allow you to be yourself. But it's not just a job that can do this. It could be a relationship, or a friendship, or the place where you live.

The good news is that you already know about being yourself. No one has to teach you. You're the world's leading expert.

What's more, you don't have to force it. In fact, if you're working hard at being yourself, you're not being yourself.

Here's what to do. Spend a few days going through your life with the phrase "If it were up to me . . ." in your head. What would you do differently if it were up to you what you had on your wall at work? If it were up to you how you spoke to clients or colleagues? If it were up to you how you dressed? If it were up to you how you did your job? If it were up to you what jobs or clients you took on? If it were up to you how you dealt with people in your family? If it were up to you how you spent your leisure time?

This last one is a good example. Let's say you're going on vacation to Hawaii. Great. But this is your vacation, and you've got to be able to say you did it your way. Maybe you want to be active the whole time. Then that's what you should do, and don't let anyone stop you. Maybe you just want to lie on the beach. That's fine too.

If you keep asking how you would do this and that differently "if it were up to me," I promise that you'll find countless pockets of freedom, as I call them. You'll be surprised at how many opportunities there are in your life for you to do it your way. Maybe you didn't bother looking for these pockets of freedom. Maybe you knew they were there but for some reason you held yourself back from taking the opportunity to do things your own way.

I'll tell you a secret about myself. Whenever I find my emotional energy running low, I find some way to say, 'Screw them all—I'm going to do what I want to do and say what I want to say, at least in one small area.' I mine one little pocket of freedom. Here's an example. I like eating a big dinner. But it's not healthy to eat late. Plus all the experts tell you to have a big breakfast. But I don't like breakfast foods. So when I'm home, I have dinner for breakfast. When you're eating eggs, I'm eating lasagna. So sue me! But it's only partly about eating in a way that works for me. Emotionally what's critical is that I've found one more little way to be myself.

But don't do what I do or what Wendy or Andrew did. That's the whole point. Be more *yourself*.

Emotional energy booster #4
Wherever you can in your life, do things your own way.

Whenever you hit a pocket of freedom and make good use of it, you'll feel like a kid let out of school on a warm spring Friday afternoon. The more pockets of freedom you take advantage of, the more energy you'll have.

Special Issue:

You, the Universe, and Your Emotional Energy

I'd like you to imagine a kind of cosmic boxing ring.

In this corner of the ring there's just you. In the other corner there's *the entire rest of the universe*. Who do you think wins that boxing match? Sorry, you lose.

Now let's change it. Suppose that in one corner of the ring there are the parts of your life that you're up against. In the other corner there's you and *the entire rest of the universe* in sync with each other. Now who do you think wins? It's your corner all the way.

The point is that the universe is filled with natural forces. If you oppose them, you exhaust yourself. No one has enough emotional energy to fight the universe. But if you align yourself with the natural forces in the universe, you link up your energy with an enormous energy source. You can never exhaust yourself.

You can think about this spiritually, practically, morally, any way you want. For example, if you're trying to help your fellow human beings and you think the universe deeply and thoroughly wants us to help one another, that profoundly adds to the emotional energy you get from trying to help people. You're on the side of the angels. You're playing for the winning team. You're going with the flow.

Whatever you do, and however you think about it, you should be feeling that what you're doing is working with and for the energy of the universe. If not, do something different.

High-energy people do specific things that work so they'll have the best possible relationship with the universe. And all the secrets here reflect this. All the secrets will quickly give you big hits of emotional energy because they'll make you feel you've got the entire universe in your corner.

Maybe the best examples of this are people such as Gandhi. Gandhi had goals and dreams and desires like all of us. But he didn't just want to win: "I win. You lose. Ha ha." He wanted what he felt the entire universe was crying out for. He wanted what he felt was the direction the universe was taking. He was hitched up not only to the world's biggest fuel supply but to the world's biggest engine. The forces Gandhi was struggling against—the entire British Empire and the ignorance of hundreds of millions of his own people—were puny by comparison.

In his later years Gandhi said that what best summed up his spiritual beliefs was contained in the first verse of the Isa Upanishad, which Gandhi himself translated as follows:

All this that we see in this great universe is permeated by God.
Renounce it and enjoy it.
Do not covet anybody's wealth or possession.

I'm going to ask you to think about these three lines very carefully, because they are very important.

The first line makes it clear why we have to heal our relationship with the universe. That's because every part is connected with every other part. Whatever God is, that's what links everything and everyone together.

And this is the only *fact* that Gandhi wants us to focus on: The universe is a force field permeated by goodness.

The rest of his core beliefs are all commands.

Now here's the really great part. The commands to renounce and not covet are both negative. They tell you what not to do. And they're basically telling you not to get too attached to transient and unimportant things.

The one positive command at the heart of Gandhi's beliefs, the one and only thing he actually urges you to do, is to enjoy life.

Now just think for a moment what that means for you specifically, today and for the rest of your life. Is there any clearer possible indication of what you need to do to heal your relationship with the universe? *Enjoy life*. And that means that you have to be yourself and feel at home in the world, because nothing, nothing is more personal to you than enjoyment.

Think about what it would do for your emotional energy if the forces you're struggling against seemed puny compared to the forces you had at your side working with you.

But everything in life, however grand, must be implemented in practical, specific ways. And that's where the secrets of high-energy people come in. They show us all exactly how to heal our relationship with the universe in ways we all can do.

I had no ideological or spiritual bias or agenda in my research. And yet all the secrets I've discovered help us in one way or another to renounce what's unimportant, to renounce what we can't control, to heal our relationship with the universe by making it a place that feels more healthful and nurturing, and to enjoy the gift of life. Amazing! Ancient wisdom and modern science converge.

5

See Yourself Having Emotional Energy

Emotional Energy Booster #5

Diagnostic Question #5

Are you in the habit of visualizing yourself living your life with emotional energy?

*   A no answer to this question means that this secret will give you a big boost of emotional energy.*

Visualization is a technique for getting better at doing something by mentally seeing yourself do that thing. And I used to think it was hogwash. I'm such a hard-nosed person. I thought people learned a lot more by *doing* than by visualizing. But I talked to successful baseball players, golfers, and tennis pros about how they kept their emotional energy up under difficult circumstances. And they kept talking about visualizing as an essential part of their preparation.

So I've changed my mind. I was wrong. Visualization works, and it specifically works unusually well to increase emotional energy.

Seeing Yourself with Emotional Energy

Here's what one guy who was a shortstop for a baseball team said. (For people like me who don't really know what a shortstop is, he's the guy who stands near second base and the batter hits balls to him hard, and he has to try to catch the ball and then make a fast, accurate throw to one of the other guys standing near one of the bases. The point is that he's under a lot of pressure and what he does makes a big difference.)

Hector, 28: "You hear the sports announcers talk about a routine play. I hate that. I think that's death for a shortstop. You can't think that any play is routine. You gotta think that anything can happen, because that's all that ever happens, crazy stuff. The ball can come at you a thousand different ways. And then you have to get rid of it and make an accurate throw even if you're lying flat on your back. And if you make one little mistake, you're the goat.

"You've got to be mentally prepared. It's like inside you feel ready. You're there. You're not afraid. You're kind of looking forward to whatever they have to throw at you.

"To get into this place I have to visualize. I didn't use to know what that meant. I just thought it was crazy stuff some sports psychologist came up with. But now I see that it's the one thing that makes the biggest difference between my having a good day and my having a bad day.

"Here's what I do. I like to do this lying in bed before I go to sleep when there's a game the next day. I picture myself standing at my position to the right of second base. There I am looking at the batter. The pitcher winds and delivers. The batter connects. Then I visualize whatever I feel like. A hot grounder hit right to me. A line drive to my right. A shot to the second baseman when there's a guy on first so I have to cover the bag. Whatever. A million possibilities.

"I don't visualize success, whatever that means. I just visualize myself getting the job done. I mean, if there's a grounder, you have to see yourself looking the ball right into your glove. If you're going to throw to first, you visualize yourself taking that extra split second to settle down and get a good grip on the ball so you don't throw it over the first baseman's head.

"I mean, you just see yourself being the way you'd like to be. It's no big deal. But when I don't do it, my game suffers and I feel weak inside."

All the Best People Do It

If visualizing yourself dealing effectively with whatever it is you're going to have to deal with worked for Hector and so many other athletes, it would have to work for other people. And it did, in ways I never would have predicted. Imagine my surprise at discovering that surgeons visualized themselves performing an operation the day before the big event. Pilots visualized themselves handling a variety of critical situations. Salespeople visualized meeting with clients.

The key wasn't visualizing the moment of success. It was visualizing yourself doing a good job dealing with whatever you had to deal with.

You can probably guess where I'm going with this. It turns out, much to my surprise, that *people with emotional energy visualized themselves having a lot of energy*. At night or first thing in the morning, anticipating the day to come, they would see themselves going through their day filled with an inner state of high energy. They would see themselves acting and reacting the way people do when they feel happy and hopeful and dynamic.

This is amazingly useful for people who are filled with emotional fatigue. Imagine this: You give yourself energy by seeing yourself with energy.

If you're not used to doing this, here's a very helpful hint. Let's say you're lying in bed getting ready to go to sleep. Start by seeing whatever it is you're going to have to handle the next day that might be hard for you in your present state of low energy. Now here's the trick. The first thing you do is see yourself handling this situation the way you think you would in your current emotionally exhausted state. Don't spend too much time here, but see that image of yourself doing whatever you do in a flat, gloomy, uncreative way. You need this, because it gives you a baseline, a reference point against which to do the more positive visualization. It makes positive visualizing much easier.

Then see yourself handling the situation as if you're filled with hope and spunk and vim and vigor. Just see yourself with emotional energy. Don't worry about the ultimate outcome. For example, if you're visualizing yourself having more energy during a job interview, don't waste a second visualizing the interviewer leaping out from behind the desk and offering you your dream job. Instead, see yourself leaning forward in your chair during the interview, smiling, talking in a bright way, sounding confident about yourself, feeling happy when you're asked tough questions.

You just need to see yourself coping and dealing in a new energetic way. I understand. Right now you may not feel you have all that much energy. But you're going to visualize what you'd do if you had tons.

Don't worry. You're not under any obligation. The next day, having done all this wonderful visualization, you don't have to act in any particular way. You just have to do your best. But I promise you that having given yourself the gift of basically imagining yourself acting with emotional energy, it will make a big difference in what you do in reality.

Rachel, 37: "This is a tough business, and it's particularly tough for women. And I've been doing it for a long time. I'm a local television newswoman. No, I don't anchor. Actually, I mostly go out and interview politicians and locally prominent people.

"At some point a whole bunch of stuff got to me. I mean, there's the fact that everyone you interview is either lying to you or using you. And I'm thinking my bosses are just waiting around for an opportunity to fire me. And then a couple of years ago I married this great guy who's a very successful surgeon, and I think he'd be ecstatic if I quit my job and stayed home to take care of him. I never wanted to do that, but as things got rough for me at work it was very tempting, and it kind of fed into my sense that what I did didn't make any difference, and that also hurt my emotional energy.

"Then a prominent local politician got into some trouble—accusations of kickbacks. His people contacted us and gave me an exclusive interview. I should've been happy, but it was really an insult. The thing is, I'd been getting so emotionally fatigued that my interviews were visibly soft and flat. I'd been a really tough gal, and then I lost it. And that politician was taking advantage of how weak I'd gotten.

"I think if the insult hadn't been so pointed, I would've laid down for this. But it got to me. Somehow I managed to decide that I had to get some energy from somewhere—pick myself up by my bootstraps, that kind of thing. I had an inspiration to go look at some old tapes of mine back when I was still full of piss and vinegar. You could see it right on camera. I was a pistol.

"It gave me an idea. For many days before my interview with State Senator Screw-up I just visualized myself interviewing him as if I were really up for it, you know, *there,* thinking my career is going to break nationally as a result of every next interview I do. I just saw myself talking to this guy, leaning forward, pressing into him, asking follow-up questions, not being afraid of his getting flop sweats.

"What a difference my preparing like that made. Everyone said the old Rachel was back. I did a great job. For the first time in a long time I'd really shown up for an interview. It felt fantastic. I guess you can think you've lost something, but if it was ever part of you, you can't ever lose it."

You Can Do It

Anyone can do what Rachel did. It couldn't be simpler.

Emotional energy booster #5
Give yourself energy by visualizing yourself
having emotional energy.

Maybe you've put on weight and you've just gotten fired, and now you have to go to a cousin's wedding where your whole family will be. You're so down you don't want to go. Okay. But you can see yourself in your mind's eye talking to Uncle Dave and Cousin June the way you would if you had a ton of energy. You can see yourself walking into the room with energy. And if you do, it will make an enormous difference.

If you're stuck anywhere in your life, you can do what Rachel did. See yourself tackling what you have to tackle, but tackling it filled with energy. If you have to, remember back to a time when you used to have energy. And imagine how the person you were then would have tackled it.

If you're really stuck and in a place where you can't remember ever having had any emotional energy, think about some actor who symbolizes for you the emotional energy you feel you lack. Picture Julia Roberts or Tom Hanks or whoever walking into that wedding reception. Picture one of them talking to Uncle Dave and Cousin June.

And if you really want to give yourself a lifetime gift of energy, you can conduct this little visualization exercise every night before you go to sleep. We all have a clue about what we're going to face the next day. And it's certainly better to visualize than to lie around worrying. So just see yourself facing the coming day with emotional energy, and you'll have more emotional energy when you go through that day.

6

Do Something *Really* New

Emotional Energy Booster #6

Think about the best day you had in the past week. How would you like
to live that day over and over for the rest of your life? If you're like most
people, you're not wild about that. In fact, even if it was a *great* day, it's
nauseating to think about it being endlessly repeated. And this points to a
truth: We have a deep hunger for something new. For most of us, that
hunger is justified by the fact that there's very little new in our lives.

This has a huge impact on our emotional energy. A life with little *new*
in it is like a tire with a slow leak. It may not make a difference all at once,
but the emotional energy will eventually leak out of it. You've got to do
something new to stop up the leak and fill up again with emotional
energy.

Diagnostic Question #6

Do you do something really new at least once a month?
A **no** *answer to this question means that this secret will give you a big boost of emotional energy.*

Why aren't people doing new things all the time?

Here's the problem, and I'm as guilty as most. First, we're busy. Second, we've created a good-enough routine and we're reluctant to shake it up. Third, we've tried new things in the past and they haven't always worked out. Fourth, we don't quite know what new things to do.

I've made these excuses myself. This is a way most of us are pretty conservative. And so we get stuck. We need to do something new. But we feel we can't.

Newness Is a Need

I'm here to tell you that it's a lot easier to do something new than you might think, and a lot more vital to your health and happiness.

Maura, 36: "I'm a waitress at a steak house, plus I do catering jobs when I can. My husband owns a small auto body shop, and we have two sons, eight and ten. For most of our married life it's all been about working hard and paying bills. Always having to think about money gets you locked in. If Ed or me got sick, forget about it—we'd be in big trouble.

"We're like millions of people who've gotten ourselves into a place that's just good enough and just precarious enough where we pray nothing changes. Well, beware of getting what you pray for. It was always the same routine in the morning, my getting Ed and the kids out. Then you do chores and shopping. Then you get dinner started, the kids come home, and around the time when Ed comes home I'm off to the restaurant. It's like a dance routine. Everyone has to know their steps.

"And then I got to the point where I just didn't want to get out of bed. I wasn't tired, mind you. Frankly, I don't have a very hard life. And I sort of take good care of myself. It was more like, God, you look ahead and nothing ever, ever is going to change. Because nothing *can* change.

"I was also having fantasies about walking away from the whole thing. I kept telling myself I would never do that, and of course I really couldn't, but I'd hear about towns in the news—an explosion in Cheyenne, Wyoming, or a teachers' strike in Baton Rouge, Louisiana—and I'd be thinking 'Hmmm . . . I wonder what it's like to live there,' and I'd look on the news for a shot of people's houses, just to get a sense of what it would be like for me if I lived there. That's how bored and unhappy I was.

"But I have a lifeline. Sometimes I get together with a few ladies and we talk about everything, you know, like they do on *Sex and the City,* except without the sex and without the city. And without the gorgeous clothes.

"But, good Lord, we do talk. And one day one of the ladies out of nowhere says, 'You know, sometimes I could just scream.' And we looked at her, and there was a scary kind of haunted look on her face like you were looking into a secret you weren't supposed to know about. To make a long story short, it turns out that we're all dying of boredom. And I don't mean that we're very bored. I mean that boredom is really killing us.

"So we started talking about, man, we've got to do something. Just to shake things up a little. And all these crazy ideas came out. That was the best time. Talking about all the new things we were going to do.

"Of course, no one did anything. But it got me thinking. I asked myself what most made me want to scream. It was really just my day-to-day routine. I knew it was always going to be the same. And I thought about my friend someday maybe going off the deep end, and that's what pushed me to the point where I realized I had to save my life.

"So I thought about what I could do that would be new. First I thought I could exercise. I wanted to do those classes you hear about that are kind of fun and get your whole body moving. Meet new people too. So I joined a gym in the next town. It had yoga. Imagine me doing yoga. Now that's *new*.

"Let me see, what else? I changed my look. I didn't want to look so small-town. I cut my hair short. I bought some black T-shirts. Oh, and my lady friends and I decided to take a trip to New York, see a show, go to a club, shop on Fifth Avenue—at least window-shop. Scare our husbands a little.

"You can't believe what a new thing can do for you. It's not about the thing itself. I mean, come on, who cares if you change your clothes? But it's like you're saying, 'Hey, I can rescue myself.' You know that scene at the end of *An Officer and a Gentleman* when Richard Gere comes into the factory and picks up Debra Winger and carries her away? I don't want to sound like a feminist, but we've really got to feel we can do that for *ourselves*. If someone's going to change my life, it's going to be me.

"So while I was busy doing new things, I quit my job. It's not that we don't need the money. I'd been waitressing because my catering wasn't exactly taking off. But I realized maybe my catering isn't taking off because of the time I spend waitressing. Where I am now is trying to get more catering jobs. I've taken out ads. Called places. I've talked to my minister about being available for weddings. It's scary. But I've gotten some jobs. I'm in a world of new things. It's exciting."

We learn a lot from Maura. When you're stuck in a routine, it's terrible for your energy. It runs down, like an old-fashioned clock that someone's forgotten to wind. Tell yourself, "If my energy's low, it's probably because I'm stuck in a routine, and so I need to do something new."

Emotional energy booster #6
Do something new.

Doing *something* new is the catalyst. What we learn from Maura (and countless people like Maura) is that it doesn't really matter what you do that's new, and it doesn't have to be something big. It may be better that it isn't something big, because that can be scary and difficult.

The key, I've learned, is this: If you wouldn't ordinarily do it, it's new enough for you. Eat a new food. Eat an old food prepared in a new way. Drive home a new way. Wear socks that are a new color for you. Do one new thing the next time you have sex. Go to the bookstore and buy a new kind of book. Listen to a new kind of music. Go to the florist and ask them to put together a little bouquet with some new and exotic flowers.

I know a secret about you. You've already been working on this. Deep down you've been hatching fantasies of new things you want to do. You already, on some level, know what you want to do. So take it off the back burner. Do it now. New things give big hits of emotional energy fast.

Special Issue:

First Aid When Your Emotional Energy Crashes

It happens. Suddenly you find yourself discouraged, unable to make an effort, feeling everything is meaningless, feeling your own personal mixture of sadness, anger, and fear. You're suddenly dropped in a pit of emotional exhaustion.

Lots of times this happens for a reason. Maybe you just got fired. Maybe you just got dumped. Maybe a big chain store just opened up near the small shop you've been struggling to keep going. Maybe a tornado just picked up your house and blew it away.

Sometimes, though, it's just that the normal junk we put up with every day finally gets to us. Your boss was a jerk. Okay. You found out your boyfriend has been talking to his old girlfriend. Okay. You see that you've put on ten pounds. Okay. So far you're still able to cope. Then you discover that your elderly cat's kidneys are failing, and suddenly you can't deal with anything anymore. It's the straw that broke the camel's back.

And sometimes your emotional exhaustion seems to come out of nowhere.

If you do nothing, you can suffer and stay stuck for a long time. Maybe you'll actually make things worse for yourself.

But you're not helpless. I've discovered that there are ten first-aid remedies that work to stop the crash and bring you out of it fast. None of this will permanently increase your emotional energy (that's what the secrets are for!), but like all good first aid, it will bring you to the point where you can feel good enough to start making things better for yourself.

So here's what to do when your emotional energy suddenly crashes.

1. Buy yourself something that you find beautiful or uplifting or delightful. Or ask someone who cares about you to buy you something like this. You know how when a crash victim goes into the emergency room they immediately start an IV? Well, something beautiful or uplifting, like flowers, is a kind of emotional IV when our emotional energy has crashed. Flowers are particularly magical because they deliver a sense of hope and beauty and a belief that life is filled with wonderful things and the possibility of endless new beginnings. You could also get yourself a book or a poster or a CD. It's easy. It's fast. This is a great place to start your first aid.

2. If your emotional energy has crashed, your physical energy needs to help you out. So immediately do things to take care of your physical energy. Get a lot of rest. Eat a lot of protein. Force yourself to exercise, even if that only means going for long walks. (Read the Appendix, "The *Physical* Energy Factor," for a complete list of physical energy builders.)

3. Throw yourself into your work. I hate clichés, and this was one I had to test. Everyone says that when something bad happens to you that gets you down, the best thing to do is keep busy, particularly doing the work you have to do. And if you don't have something to do, this is when you need to get busy with something. Well, it's true. People who get back their emotional energy the fastest are precisely the ones who keep busy, and people who sit back, nursing their emotional wounds, stay stuck longer.

4. Immediately do little things you know will make you happy. Do your best to remember back to things you've done that have made you happy. Like what? Maybe there are certain movies you're a fan of. Rent a couple of them. Maybe there's someplace out in nature you enjoy being. Go there. Maybe you always cheer up when you hear a certain kind of music. Make sure you listen to it. Maybe there's a person in your life who always lifts your spirits. Get together with that person.

Whether or not any of the things that have made you happy in the past make sense to you right now, do them anyway. If you can't think of anything, ask someone who knows you well to remind you of what you've done that you've enjoyed.

Hopefully, though, you're lucky enough to be reading these words before you've fallen into an emotional energy crash. So *right now* think of three things to do that always make you happy. Write them on a piece of paper. This is your emergency kit for whenever your emotional energy suddenly crashes. Then when you need it, don't ask questions—just do them. The important thing is that even if you don't feel like doing them, you have to do them anyway.

5. Find someone smart that you trust, and talk to this person about your emotional energy collapse—why it happened, what you can do for yourself right now, why you should feel hopeful about the future. This is the time to get real support from someone who's able to give it. Whatever you do, make sure you don't feel alone. It doesn't matter if this person is a friend or a professional. Just make sure this person is someone who can and will encourage you and direct you. There's hope, and you need someone to help you find it.

6. Have appropriate expectations for yourself right now. Say something like this to yourself: "I'm going to have a couple of days of feeling *really* lousy, a couple of days of *sort of* feeling lousy, and then I'll start getting bored and distracted with being down and I'll find I'm starting to come out of this." It gives you emotional energy to know that this too shall pass.

Now you know that what you're going through is temporary. You'll be okay. You can be patient with yourself. You can know that you can afford to focus on taking care of yourself. You can see why it's worthwhile not to make any big, life-changing decisions.

7. Give yourself some solitude. This would be a perfect time to go camping, for example. Spend time alone in the middle of nature, on a beach or in a park. Don't be alone in a depressing place. But solitude in a beautiful place—it might just be sitting alone in a place of worship—accelerates the healing process.

8. *Identify what you're afraid of.* Usually part of the reason your emotional energy has crashed is fear. Only when you identify your fear can you prevent it from controlling you. You're almost certainly plunged into exhaustion because you don't think you can deal with whatever it is you're afraid of. You're suddenly so far down because you don't think you can get back up to where you need to go. You have disaster scenarios in your head. You're wrestling with visions of how impossible things are.

But when you specify your fear—rather than living in a wordless state of emotional collapse—you're better able to answer your fear with a voice of reason and common sense. Whatever it is you're afraid of, there are always two great solutions. One, you can see how unlikely it is that what you're afraid of will ever happen. Two, you can do things to protect yourself or take care of yourself. Either solution will make you feel much better.

9. *Take one small step toward making your life better.* You don't know what to do? It doesn't matter. Don't rack your brain. It doesn't have to be a brilliant idea. Make a guess about something you could do that would have a good chance of making your life better rather than worse.

Here are just a few possible suggestions. Join a health club. Buy a new electronic toy. Go get a really good haircut. Hire someone to clean your house. Throw out a bunch of junk that's been cluttering up one of your rooms. Get a stack of good books from the library and read only the one that you're really interested in. Buy some kind of clothing that you haven't bought for yourself in a long time. Call up an old friend you haven't been in touch with. Call a local college and ask them to send you a catalogue of extension courses.

But don't just sit there. Do something. Do it now. Everything you do now that doesn't make your life worse will make your life better and will make you feel much better. Action is the answer.

10. *Reread this book.* I designed *The Emotional Energy Factor* to be

a lifetime resource. As you and your life change, you never know which secret will prove to be the perfect remedy. So if your emotional energy has just crashed, there's almost certainly another emotional energy booster in this book that will feel right to you and that will kick-start you toward regaining your energy.

7

What Are You Looking Forward To?

Emotional Energy Booster #7

Most kids are filled with the sense of something wonderful to look forward to. Grandma's coming on Saturday! In two weeks it'll be my birthday! It's Christmas in ten days! Next week there's a school trip, school play, or just plain old end of school! I'm going to sleep-away camp! Bobby asked me out! Sally said she'd date me! I'm getting a bra, a car, a job!

Be honest. Do you have wonderful things to look forward to *now*?

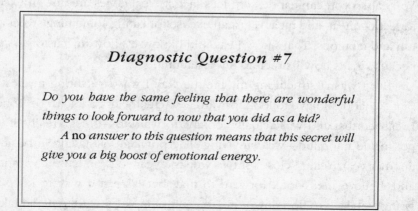

Diagnostic Question #7

Do you have the same feeling that there are wonderful things to look forward to now that you did as a kid?

A **no** *answer to this question means that this secret will give you a big boost of emotional energy.*

Lots of us can say that on balance, being fair, we have a good life. No reason to feel enormously sorry for ourselves. Still, duties and responsibilities fill our days. Every life is to some degree a tough desert that you have to trudge through. It's normal and we can handle it, but it still can sometimes feel like a desert. Trudge, trudge, trudge. Weekend? Yes, but there are always chores. Too often weekends feel routine. Vacations? They're great, but too often they're not all that special.

Special Treats

There has to be an oasis. Something to dream about, something to look forward to luxuriating in when you get there. But for too many of us it's too much desert and not enough dessert.

Jimmy, 44: "I wish people wouldn't assume my life is one big party. I'm the chef/owner of a highly praised restaurant. Big deal. Here's what my life is *really* like. With the debt I had to take on to start this place, I'm sure as hell not making money. Day to day, my life is just work, work, work, pressure, pressure, pressure. What every day feels like is . . . well, imagine the captain of the *Titanic* was also a one-armed paperhanger. Something like that.

"The one thing that's kept me going is my belief that dessert is king. You eat so you can eat dessert, let's face it. Vegetables are just an excuse for eating meat, and meat is just an excuse for eating something sweet and fun and fabulous. That's how I eat, and I know it's how my customers eat, because that's how I structure my restaurant.

"But I wasn't structuring my life the way I was structuring my restaurant. What did I have to look forward to? Actually, not a lot. To be honest, I realized that all I was actually looking forward to—I mean really, if you got inside my mind—was surviving. The privilege of staying in business another year. Yeah, I close for two weeks a year so I can have a 'vacation,' and, believe me, I look forward to that, but it's just a way to keep me going. A beach to flop down on. You sort of look forward to it and take it for granted all at the same time. It's more like it'll kill you not to have it than that it gets you all excited knowing that you're going to have it.

"On Fridays this one group usually gets together at the restaurant, and late one night they invited me to sit down and join them. 'To take a load off,' as they put it. I was pretty much done, so I did. They were mostly men and women in their thirties and forties who taught and did research at the local veterinary school. I knew they worked hard. And they started talking about these really special things they had to look forward to.

"They had just as many burdens and responsibilities as I did. They had just as much reason to keep looking over their shoulders. But it was like they understood that at some point you have to let go of all that grim sense of duty and put something magical out there in the future for yourself.

"Like what? One guy was talking about sailing a small boat across the Atlantic. Now that's a big deal. One woman talked about buying a horse. Another talked about having a baby. One couple talked about driving cross-country together using just the back roads. And one guy talked about taking some time out and learning how to make violins.

"I could see how much energy they got from whatever it was that they looked forward to. None of it was a big deal in the grand scheme of things. It was just that for those people, they had something special in the future that they knew was going to happen. And it made them very happy.

"And it was so clear to me that these vets had dessert to look forward to in their lives. Something special. That was what I needed. And then it hit me. I could never find anything that would justify taking time away from the restaurant. So I never had anything special to look forward to. Like something that for me would be a big treat, traveling. But then I found a loophole, I guess. I'd travel and visit the kitchens of restaurants around the world. Maybe the chef would be the friend of a friend. Maybe it would be a restaurant I'd read about and admired. Maybe they'd have a style of cooking I'd wanted to learn about.

"It turned out to be very exciting. It's like when you get to take a tax deduction on a trip you take for pleasure. Except in my case I could justify professionally something that, let's face it, was just a lot of fun for me.

"The surprising part is how much I've enjoyed looking forward to my little trips. There's always some delicious experience laying in wait for me in the not-too-distant future. It makes me very happy. And I have so much more to give to the restaurant now. It's funny how that works."

Life is filled with mysteries until you understand how emotional energy works, and then a lot of things get clear. Jimmy was a hardworking guy, seemingly maxed out. Then he *added* something to his life, and yet he ended up with more energy. How could that be?

How Better Futures Make Better Presents

You get fuel from having something special to look forward to. It's the carrot in a world of sticks. But most of us don't have all that many things we really look forward to in the sense that they make us feel excited. But when you do have something like that, it keeps you going.

The key is your sense of anticipation. *You don't even have to actually do the thing you're looking forward to.* Just the fact that you have something to look forward to, somewhere in the future, is enough. Of course it can't feel too remote. It's got to feel doable in the not-too-distant future.

Emotional energy booster #7
Always have something special to look forward to.

For example, I have a close friend—my oldest friend, in fact—who lives in a different city. We rarely see each other. One day we decided we're going to take a vacation together. Just the two of us, no husbands. This is definitely a big deal for us. We're both very busy, so it can't happen this year, but it's sitting there waiting for us, a special oasis of anticipation.

I have lots of things in my life that I look forward to. But everything other than that trip feels normal. I expect to have those things. It's more like I'd feel cheated if I didn't have them. But that little trip with my friend—that's a real dessert. Unnecessary. Unexpected. Not huge. But special and unique.

By the way, going on a special trip turned out to be the number-one choice of people when I asked them what they had to look forward to that gave them the most emotional energy.

By giving yourself something special to look forward to, you let go of the burden of feeling tied down by routine. You stop experiencing your own life as a kind of treadmill that you're trapped on. Everyone who has something terrific to look forward to feels lighter and freer.

It doesn't have to be a big deal. It doesn't have to cost much money. It doesn't have to be special to anyone but you. But it has to feel special. And it has to be outside of your day-to-day, year-to-year routine. If you have something like this already, you know it. If you don't, you need it.

These Are a Few of My Favorite Things

Okay, so you need to have something special to look forward to in your life. You also should have something special to look forward to every day. Maybe not something enormously special. But definitely a treat. Quick, tell me—what treat are you looking forward to today? You should always have an answer to this question, every single day, as a permanent antidote to emotional exhaustion.

It's easy and fun to come up with a treat to look forward to every day. Just make a list of the favorite things that you've done that have given you emotional energy.

Don't turn your special-things list into a to-do list. This is no more a to-do list than eating dessert is a daily chore. This is a wish list. Even better, this is a kind of pleasure map to your life. Every life is filled with peaks and valleys. But scattered throughout every life are bits of buried pleasure. Your list of the things that give you energy is a map to where the pleasure is buried in your life.

Here you are, parched of emotional energy. And yet there's an underground river of pleasure you can tap into whenever you want by doing things you enjoy! I call that the opposite of a chore. I call that a gift.

And all you have to do is think of it. When you're falling asleep, when you're driving to work, instead of thinking about stuff that's no fun to think about, think about what you could do that would be a treat.

And the emotional energy will flow in.

When it comes to the body, we know that people don't exercise because they're healthy. People are healthy because they exercise. Energy is all about what you do, not who you are. So in the same way, people don't feel they have things to look forward to because they have emotional energy. People have emotional energy because they give themselves things to look forward to.

8

Why Should a Barrel Full of Monkeys Have More Fun Than You?

Emotional Energy Booster #8

One of the themes that runs through this book is the idea that you don't have to make big moves to get a big payback in energy. Some of the best things you can do require only slight attitudinal shifts. And that makes sense. It takes energy to get energy—you have to drive to the gas station, walk to the refrigerator—so what we all want is the biggest boost in energy for the smallest investment.

That's where fun comes in. Fun isn't something you do. Fun is the *way* you do something.

Watch a kid trapped in a no-fun zone. He might be in school on a warm Friday afternoon. His head's resting on his arm, his eyelids are drooping, he can barely hold his pencil. Suddenly the three o'clock bell rings. The kid is boosted out of the no-fun zone straight into the fun zone. And watch his energy. It zooms. What happened? Fun.

You can see this going on at work. You're in the middle of a boring conversation in the break room. Someone walks in with a juicy bit of gossip. Suddenly a hot current of energy starts flowing through the veins of everyone. Fun jump-started everyone's energy.

Fun Aerates Energy

Fun changes everything. Fun is to energy what breathing is to life. Without it you asphyxiate.

I once made this experiment. I did therapy with my patients exactly as I'd been doing it. I only made one tiny change. For one week at the beginning of every session I said, "What we're going to do today isn't going to be much fun." The following week at the beginning of every session I said: "Let's have some fun today." I couldn't believe the enormous difference it made. The sessions with the no-fun intro were blah. The sessions with the fun intro had more commitment, involvement, and creativity. Emotional energy was much higher when fun was expected.

Since then I've tried to find a way (when appropriate) not just to inject fun in my clinical work but to make it clear that that's what I'm doing. And I do that because it gives emotional energy, and emotional energy makes everything we do more productive and more satisfying.

Diagnostic Question #8

Would you say that there's really not much fun in your everyday life?

A **yes** *answer to this question means that this secret will give you a big boost of emotional energy.*

Fun Is Totally Doable

The great thing about this secret is how much energy you get from making a very slight shift.

Emotional energy booster #8
Just say to yourself: "Today, I'll be just a little less serious,
a little less obsessively goal-oriented. I'll try to have
a little more fun doing whatever I do."

People sometimes make one of two objections to this. They might say, "But I'm not such a fun person." Or they say, "You don't know my work/ my life/my situation. If you did, you'd know there's no way to have fun here."

I understand. Some of us are more serious than others. Many of us are in situations that demand the utmost seriousness. All this is a given. But what do you think I'm asking you to do? Change yourself or your life? Absolutely not. Do you think I'm telling you how to have fun? Absolutely not.

I'm just bringing you news from the front lines: Everyone, regardless of context, can push the boundaries a little and can have a little more fun, however you'd define fun. Even the most serious person in the most serious job can have just a little more fun. And if he does, he'll have *a lot* more emotional energy.

Thomas, 46: "I really hate the stereotypes people have of funeral directors. We're just ordinary people doing an important job. Admittedly, dealing with death is unusual, but I really don't think *we're* all that unusual. Besides, if you ask any of us, we'll say we don't really deal with death as much as we deal with living people and their living needs.

"Obviously, though, this is a profession that requires a certain seriousness. Now, here's what happened to me. I took our business over from my father when he retired. I wanted to—don't get me wrong. But you do have this sense that maybe you wouldn't have chosen to be a funeral director if your father had owned a shoe store. Here I am, though, and of course my father always trained me to deal with people with sympathy and dignity, to help them through a very tough period in their lives, the loss of a loved one.

"It all started feeling very oppressive—all this sympathy and dignity I was putting out. My life started splitting in two. I was very serious with our clients. And I would joke around a lot when I wasn't on duty. But the more serious I was with our clients, the more I felt discontented and resentful. It started feeling more and more emotionally exhausting to face a grieving relative.

"I found myself talking about getting out of the business. That scared me. I've made a good living here, and honestly, I'm one of the good guys. My profession needs people like me. I wondered if I could give myself new energy for my work. Then I realized I needed to have more fun on the job. I'd thought this is the last profession in the world for fun. But I realized I'd better find a way or else. You don't clown around with someone in mourning, obviously. But I did find there were a lot of little things I could do.

"For example, it was a lot better for all of us, me and the clients, if I asked them to tell me about the deceased. What kind of a person was he? What did he do for fun? What gave him pleasure? What was he good at? What interesting things happened to him? That's not clowning around. But it's a hell of a lot more fun than only talking about casket options.

"I found that people were so eager to open up and talk about positive things about the person who'd just died that it stopped being so heavy for all of us. You know, people who are in the first stages of mourning don't want you to minimize what they're dealing with, but they don't need a stranger to make it too serious either. Mourning is very private, and if I can provide something of a respite, they're very grateful.

"Of course, the biggest impact was on me. I said to myself, 'I can have fun at work.' It was like I'd flipped a switch. To be honest, the changes I made were pretty small. We still had to talk about the price of caskets. But the change in my attitude was pretty big. And that made all the difference."

Harriet, 34: "They told me the army was like society except more so, and they were right. There's more opportunity for women in the army today than almost anywhere else. But you know the old idea that a woman's got to be twice as good as a man? In the army you've got to be four times as good. That's true for me. I have reached the rank of captain and command a training unit in an area of army intelligence. We train enlisted personnel and new officers. It's serious work. When intelligence does its job, the battle's over a lot faster. When we don't, a lot of our people die. That's about as stark as it gets.

"I came out of West Point extremely gung ho. There was the issue of women in combat, and I wanted to push the envelope. What happened for me was that my work got real boring real fast. I never thought that would happen. But there's a lot of routine. The main thing, I realize now, is how grim I was about it all. You know, I was going to be the most squared-away junior commanding officer in the army. Definitely senior officer material.

"Meanwhile I'm starting to not look forward to my days. And I'm finding out from some of my evaluations that, yeah, I'm pretty organized, but as a leader I'm kind of blah. That was a shock. What am I supposed to do, put on a show? Clearly I had to make an adjustment. I started looking around at the leaders I respected. Senior officers. Sergeants too. And what I noticed was that they were all more relaxed than I was. It was like they were saying they were entitled to command.

"And how did they show that? Yeah, of course there's that confident, squared-away quality, but I noticed that a lot of them had a glint of a sense of humor in dealing with subordinates. It was as if a little joke or a little piece of sarcasm or a little, I guess, playfulness said loud and clear that you were relaxed, you weren't sweating, and you weren't afraid. You didn't have to push because it wouldn't occur to anyone not to jump to your suggestions.

"That's been the knock on women, that we're too serious. Speaking for myself, I decided to lighten up. I'm a country girl. I have brothers. We knew how to have fun and still get the job done. So I decided to kid the guys and not take myself so seriously. It's not worth it if I'm not having some fun.

"I changed, and two things happened. One, I'm concentrating on my work more. I'm not wishing I were somewhere else. Two, I'm a more effective officer. I saw that right away. I saw it most in guys being able to listen to me more. That's key, being listened to. And when I'm having a little fun on the job, I get listened to."

Chuck, 29: "I'm a golf pro trying to nail down my position on the permanent tour. It's constant pressure, every hole, every shot. A couple of bad tournaments and I'm gone. And that, of course, is the key—how to deal with pressure. We're all talented. We all have good technique. It comes down to how you deal with the pressure.

"I noticed that most of my problems are on the back nine. Somehow I was losing focus. I tried to concentrate harder, and my concentration fell apart even more. I didn't want to turn into a head case. But I was exhausted inside, and the heaviness of it all was killing me.

"Then I read about this great cello player, Pablo Casals, and he's pressing his fingers up and down on these tight, heavy strings, and how does he prevent himself from getting exhausted? Here's how. No matter how fast a passage he plays, when he picks up a finger he relaxes it, even if for only a split second. That was it. Concentration is a muscle. The more you need to use it, the more you need to relax it, otherwise it gets all used up. And I'd be out there on the course tense with concentration for every single minute of eighteen holes, and then I'd try to keep that up for three days of play.

"So I said screw it. Yeah, concentrate when you're lining up a shot. Focus when you're hitting. But once the ball leaves the club face, have fun till the next shot. What does that mean? You know, kibitz a little with the caddy. Joke with a spectator. Kid one of the other players. Play loose.

"It worked. Having fun didn't spoil my concentration. It was what I thought—by having more fun, it was like I gave my concentration a rest, and so it had more energy for getting down to business when I called on it. What can you say? A happy golfer is a good golfer. It was certainly true for me."

Thomas, Harriet, and Chuck are serious people doing work that requires serious attention. But emotional exhaustion was sabotaging their effectiveness and their enjoyment. All they did, in a way that felt comfortable and appropriate, was inject an attitude of having a little bit more fun. And that liberated a lot of energy.

To do this you just have to make a decision. In your own way you're going to make your life more fun. And not just at work. If there's any part of your life where you'd like to have more emotional energy, have a little more fun there and you will.

Special Issue:

Emotional Energy and Weight Loss

The emotional energy *diet*? You bet. It's terrific. And it may be just what you've been looking for.

What's the real reason for eating? To give ourselves physical energy. But lots of times our energy feels low even though our bodies have all the physical energy we need. It's *emotional* energy that's lacking.

Many of us have been here. But then all the food in the world won't satisfy. Yet we eat anyway, because it's hard to distinguish the real reasons for feeling low energy. Food is an easy answer. This is why so many of us overeat and get fat. We're using food as a source of emotional energy.

This points to a wonderful solution to the difficulties so many of us have had losing weight.

Vi, 56: "I've been a weight-loss counselor for, what is it? Twenty-four years now. And I've seen it all. I don't care what the ads say. It's tough to lose weight. And, to be honest, it's been a battle for me too, sometimes a losing battle. As I like to put it, if you want to be thin, you have to be born that way or prepared to fight for it.

"But here's what I see when people come back to me week after week and talk about why they had trouble. 'I was bad this week,' they say. Why? Well, sometimes it's because there were three birthday parties and a wedding that week. But most of the time what you hear is 'I was bad because I was lonely,' 'I wasn't having any fun,' 'I was sad,' 'I was bored,' 'I was stressed out,' 'I was nervous,' 'I didn't have any good things happening to me.'

"Food is one kind of fuel. Sometimes, though, the kind of fuel we need the most is emotional. Whatever puts people in a weakened emotional state, bang—they turn to food. This is just my guess, but I'd say that for every ten pounds you're overweight, eight of those pounds came from feeding emotional fatigue.

"When did I put on the most weight? It's interesting. It wasn't after my divorce. By that point I was pretty much relieved and looking forward to whatever was going to come next. But I put on the most weight in that long dark period when our marriage was ending and I couldn't really face it and I didn't know what to do about it and I felt so much hopelessness and loss. So of course I ate.

"For me the divorce gave me hope, so it was a source of emotional energy. You can't get a divorce every time you need more emotional energy, but thank God you don't have to. Here's how I think of it. Food should be something you do for yourself that's healthy and feels good. If you're needing a boost emotionally, okay, fine, then you need to do something for yourself that's emotionally healthy and feels good. You totally need to feed yourself. But you don't need *food* food. You need to do something that's fun or spiritual or something that makes you feel good about yourself or something that connects you up to some kind of emotional nourishment, like talking to someone you care about.

"It's really kind of simple. Physical hunger requires physical food. Emotional hunger requires emotional food. If you satisfy each of your hungers with the appropriate kind of food, then you'll never ever be fat."

Vi said it so perfectly that it's hard for me to improve on it. So let me just underline her point. When we're trying to lose weight, we will have hungers and cravings. You have to understand that 90 percent of these hungers and cravings are real, but they are for emotional fuel, emotional energy. You really do need to take something in. You really do need something delicious in your life, or something spicy, or something sweet. But it's not food that you need to take in. It's not food that will really seem delicious to you.

If you're needing someone to say "I love you," ask for that. Don't eat ice cream. Ice cream will never make you feel loved.

If you're needing to laugh, go somewhere or to someone who will make you laugh. Don't eat cookies. They will never crack you up.

If you're needing to feel that you're doing something that helps someone else, help someone, particularly someone who will be appreciative. Don't eat another helping of pasta. That will never make you feel you're a worthwhile person.

If you're needing to feel young, do the kinds of things you did when you really were young, even if the "days of your youth" were only yesterday. Don't eat junk food. It's not the food you ate when you were young that gave you your youthfulness.

If you're needing to feel creative, do something creative. Write the worst poem in the world. Get out your colored Magic Markers and make the worst picture in the world. But don't eat cake. There's absolutely no way to eat cake that will make you feel creative.

If you're needing to tell an obnoxious person to get lost, do it, by all means. But don't eat a pizza instead. You'll just feel you're being an obnoxious person to yourself.

If you're uncertain about your future, do one tiny thing to make your future better. But don't just open up a jar of peanut butter and start eating off the spoon. The only future that will give you is a fat one.

If you're needing to talk to God, do it. There's no waiting line. But don't waste money stuffing yourself at an expensive restaurant. The greatest chef in the world may think he's God, but he isn't.

If you're needing to listen to your child talk to you, go to your child and listen. But don't stuff yourself with candy. All the candy in the world won't satisfy you.

If you're needing to dip your feet in an ocean or a lake, do it. Or go to a swimming pool, or take a bath. But an ocean of food in you won't give you what a real ocean around you will give you.

All this is good news. It means that there are so many ways you can give yourself more emotional energy. And every time you do, you'll have a victory in your campaign to lose weight.

This is the emotional energy diet. I'll make you a promise. If you eat food only to satisfy your need for physical nourishment and your physical hunger, and if you make sure that you follow the secrets in this book to feed your need for emotional energy, *you will lose weight*. And think of how much emotional energy *that* will give you.

9

Don't Get Stuck
with Your Losses

Emotional Energy Booster #9

We all have aches in the archives of our lives. Everyone, no matter how happy he or she seems, has a past studded with losses and regrets. There were mistakes and missed opportunities. We've all had things taken away from us that create a sadness that's hard to shake.

The fact that you feel this keenly means you have a heart and a conscience. Your life matters to you. You and I really don't want to have anything to do with people who aren't shaken and colored by the rough experiences they've gone through.

But from the point of view of our emotional energy, a sense of loss by itself is dead weight. When you're burdened by feelings of regret and missed opportunity, what you're really talking about is a kind of mourning, but worse. With real mourning you go through a process where there's light at the end of the tunnel. No one has much energy a day or a week after the death of a loved one. What about a year later? Five years? By then they should have recovered their energy. If not, isn't there something wrong?

Diagnostic Question #9

Would you say, "I rarely go more than a couple of days without having feelings about one of the losses, regrets, or missed opportunities in my life"?

A **yes** *answer to this question means that this secret will give you a big boost of emotional energy.*

Loss Is a Trap

You're an energy seeker. But you may also be a truth seeker: someone for whom it's very important to discover, face, and understand the truths of your life. You may be someone who hates being in denial about the things that have happened to you and what they mean. You may hate the idea of pretending that what happened didn't happen.

I understand completely. As you'll see, I've been the same way most of my life. And that means that in a weird way I was fascinated by the losses and difficulties that lurked in my past. Lots of us are.

But this is a tragedy for our emotional energy. Whatever the truth of your past, the truth of your future is that *anyone who can't let go of loss after a reasonable amount of time is in trouble and needs help.* That's because when the sense of loss lingers past its expiration date, it starts to stink up the joint. If the sense of loss doesn't depart all by itself, you have to kick it out, or else you'll be dragged down by it. You can't have emotional energy unless you get rid of your sense of loss.

In a moment I'll show you how to do just that.

How I Dealt with Loss

I've had my share of losses. I lost my father when I was four and my parents divorced. We'd been living in a displaced-persons camp in Germany. My father went with my sister to Israel. My mother took my brother and me to New York. I didn't see my father again until I was sixteen, but we never had a real relationship. As a little refugee girl, I lost out on something many of my friends had: growing up in an American family, having a father, having relatives, having money, and having a family who knew enough about the world we lived in to guide me. These are just a few of my losses. But everyone has their own.

When you talk to people about what they've missed out on in life, you're struck by the variety of stories. One person had a cold, demanding father; another had no father at all. One person grew up in a family that could give him no education or advantages; another got a good education and then, like an idiot, utterly wasted the first fifteen years of his life after college. One person had a baby and couldn't go to college; another couldn't have a baby. Sometimes it's time that's lost, sometimes opportunity, sometimes money, sometimes hope, sometimes good memories.

I'm afraid to say that as a young woman, I clung too tightly to my losses. In a strange way they gave me a sense of safety. I thought they helped explain me to myself—my defects, my moods. They gave me an identity at times when I wasn't sure who I really was. How many of us get our sense of identity from a part of our past that's stamped with loss?

But my past also dragged me down. It was as if I'd had some broken bones but wasn't letting them heal. The thing was, I didn't know what else to do.

Then I had an experience that taught me a lot about dealing with loss.

One of the losses I carried around with me was the fact that I was the child of Holocaust survivors. I was born after the war, and nothing I went through can compare to the horrors of the Holocaust. But I had spent the first four years of my life as a refugee, first in Uzbekistan, then traveling across war-torn Eastern Europe, then in a displaced-persons camp in Germany. All those years I was surrounded by poverty, fear, and people who had suffered. I lost the first years of a normal, happy childhood.

While my mother, my brother, and I managed to get to America, as penniless immigrants we had years of struggle. All my close relatives except my parents, brother, and sister had been killed. I never knew my grandparents. I was deprived of literally dozens of aunts and uncles and God knows how many cousins.

While all of our losses are different, we all do the same thing with them. We too often focus on them, obsess about them, get lost in them, make them our lives. I got involved with organizations that promoted Holocaust awareness. I think that's important for our society, but for me it was like when you have a sore tooth and you keep poking it with your tongue just to reexperience the pain.

I was getting lost in loss.

One year—I was around thirty—I went to Israel for a special ceremony. Holocaust survivors and children of survivors came from all over the world for the first time in history to massively participate in an act of mourning and memory. At one point we all stood—thousands of us—in a line at Yad Vashem, the Israeli Holocaust memorial, so we could each place one rose on a commemorative stone.

I couldn't have predicted what happened. But during the hours-long wait to lay down my rose, surrounded by mourners and the memory of pain and loss, it hit me that enough was enough. I'd had it. You know how you get so full you literally can't eat another bite? That's what happened to me with mourning the Holocaust. I reached a point where I was finished with it.

My sense of loss was over. I'll never forget or stop caring about the real loss, but the ghosts no longer haunt me. I realize that we have a choice when it comes to a sense of loss. We can drown in it. Or we can walk out of it, dry off, and live the future we were meant to have.

On the way home from that solemn event I felt as if an enormous weight had been taken off my shoulders. It was as if megawatts of my emotional energy had been tied down by my sense of loss, and when I lost my sense of loss, all that energy was freed up again. But I was the one who liberated myself. And if I could do it, anyone could liberate themselves from a sense of loss. That gave me a new level of hope about people's ability to change that has stayed with me ever since. This is something we all can and must do.

> *Emotional energy booster #9*
> *Bad things have happened to all of us,*
> *but don't let your loss define you.*

But how exactly do you do that?

How to Let Go of Loss

In the years following this experience, I learned a lot about what works for people to stop letting losses define them. There are three routes you can take. They all work, but different routes work for different people at different times in their life. If one route doesn't work, try another, and keep trying over and over until you succeed.

Route one. Look at whatever losses, grievances, or regrets you've been carrying around, and try to let them go. This is the most direct route. Tell yourself that enough is enough. Tell yourself that the time for mourning, the time for living in the past, is over. Most of all tell yourself, "Yes, something bad happened to me. But this bad thing isn't who I am. I'm not going to let myself be defined by my hurts. And if my loss isn't me, I really don't have to pay attention to it anymore."

We do this kind of thing all the time. You don't carry around the wounds of every hurt you've ever received. Well, that means you can stop making such a big deal of the fact that your mother was mean to you or the fact that the one person you really loved walked out on you ten years ago. At some point even our own pasts become boring soap operas there's no point in tuning in to. This works for a surprising number of people.

Irene, 32: "I went through one of the worst crises of my life about four years ago. I was going with this guy—actually, he'd mostly moved in with me—and one day, out of the blue, I mean it was completely unexpected, he told me he'd met this other woman and fallen in love with her and it was all over between us. Talk about being dumped. It felt like being pushed out of an airplane. I was devastated. It's always tough to get dumped, but I'd thought of us as soul mates. I'd planned out our whole future together. Plus, to be honest, I'm kind of an okay-looking girl, nothing special, but Joe was so gorgeous and he had money, and I felt sure I'd never find anyone like him again.

"To make my sense of loss even worse, for many years I'd had these issues about my feeling that my mother didn't really like me. She adored my beautiful older sister, and she doted on my younger sister, who was very sweet and kind of sickly. But I'd always felt my mother thought of me as a disappointing annoyance. I never felt loved by her, and I couldn't let go of that.

"I did what we all do. I dragged myself through my days like a gloomy Gus, and I'd wear out my girlfriends' patience from having to listen to me go on and on about Joe. It's like I had this weight I was dragging around. I felt like a walking sob story.

"One day one of my girlfriends asked me if I was planning to be like this forever. She said, 'Because if you're going to be like this forever, let me know. But if you are going to move on, for God's sake move on. I mean, okay, Joe dumped you, but why can't you let this go? It's over. Don't think about the past. Think about the future.'

"It got to me. The past is the past, and the rest of my life lies in the future. I should let go of the past. Bad stuff happens to us, but you make yourself stop thinking about it. Don't you have better things to do than chew over what someone did to you that you can never change?"

Irene is really talking about taking route one to let go of loss. You tell yourself firmly and strongly that from now on you're not going to think about what happened to you or complain about it or obsess over it. If it pops into your head, you'll push it right out again.

And you'll do this because you're tired of carrying around your loss and you want something better. Perhaps you're wondering how it can possibly work for someone to just tell themselves to let go of some loss. But people do this all the time. Have you ever had an ugly piece of furniture that you've gotten used to, and then one day you looked at it and saw how ugly it was and immediately realized it had to go? Well, that's what some people do with their sense of loss. They realize that it's just an ugly piece of emotional furniture.

Here's another way to go down the first route for letting go of your loss. Suppose you've told yourself to let go of your loss, and you want to, but you can't. You may be smarter than you realize. You may intuitively understand that you need to get some kind of compensation before you can let go. But no one's going to pay you money. You've got to find your own compensation by looking at your life with fresh eyes. Here's what to look for.

Maybe you'll be able to let go if you can see that in fact you already have what you lost in another form. For example, as one person put it, "My father was always critical of me. And that bothers me because I wanted to feel that this person who was so important to me loved me and respected me. But I like myself now. And so do other people who care about me." It's something to think about. You can never go back and get exactly what you lost. But if you have something similar or something that compensates for it now, then that's what you focus on instead of your loss.

Maybe you can still get whatever it was that you think you lost forever. One man said, "I wasted my twenties. And that bothers me because I wanted to be further along in my life than I am right now. But if I really care about getting ahead, I can start right now and focus my energy on doing now whatever it is I think I wanted to do earlier." After all, you don't get depressed because you open the refrigerator and discover that you've run out of milk. You go to the store and buy more milk. I challenge you. This is an enormous growth opportunity. If you can find a way to get some form of what it is you feel you've lost, I promise you'll feel a surge of emotional energy.

And maybe you can live just fine without having gotten what it is you've lost. One woman said, "I screwed up the best relationship I ever had. And that bothers me because I'm afraid I'll never find true love again. But I've learned a lot, and I know myself much better, and even if I never get what I thought I wanted, I know I can be happy with whatever relationship I get now." This can be a big challenge, but it's also a gigantic opportunity for growth and a fantastic way to get tremendous emotional energy at almost zero cost. You don't actually have to do *anything*. You look at your loss. You say, "Okay, I lost it." You shrug. You move on. And you do this because you see that however real your loss was, the fact is that you don't need it now. And so to protect your emotional energy you've got to let it go.

But this route doesn't work for everyone. What if you try to let go and no matter how you look at things you can't let go? Fortunately you have other options.

Route two. One reason people have trouble letting go of loss is that they've never gone through a real mourning process, and that can cause a drain of emotional energy. If only they could mourn their loss properly once and for all, then they could let it go and move on. I'm not talking about complaining. You can't dribble it out. You've got to go for the whole shebang.

In a way I did that when I went to Israel. I'd mourned in little ways, but the huge ceremony I participated in made it possible for me to mourn in a big way—so big, in fact, that it took all the mourning out of me. This is why huge ceremonies of grief are so cleansing. This is why, for example, people in many religions are commanded to observe a strict period of mourning after a loved one's death. But at the same time most religions instruct people to move on and embrace life once the intense period of mourning is over.

In other words, maybe you can't move on because you haven't really mourned. To really mourn, you have to do something big. Like take off from work for a week and stay in bed all day every day and do nothing but cry until you have no tears left. Invite a friend to spend the weekend and spend the whole time crying until you have no more tears left. Go on a long religious retreat. Get in the car and drive aimlessly for hours, listening to sad songs on the car radio. Write a long and tear-stained good-bye letter to whoever left you or hurt you. It's put up or shut up. If you try to let go and you can't, then you're saying you're in big-time mourning. So indulge in an *experience* of big-time mourning.

Most people report that when they really let themselves go and totally indulge in a limited period of intense mourning, their sense of loss finally burns itself out. In other words, sometimes we can't let go because we haven't let ourselves squeeze out the last drop of sorrow.

If you force yourself to really mourn, you'll be able to stop mourning.

But what if even that doesn't work?

Route three. This brings you to a fork in the road. If you couldn't let go and mourning hasn't worked, you have an important choice. Hanging on to loss cripples your emotional energy. So if you still can't let go of your loss, you should face the fact that your hanging on is not about the size of your loss at all. It's about your unwillingness to embrace life. Why else would someone hold on to a shadow?

So here's your choice.

You can give yourself a good talking-to, and here's what you have to tell yourself: Everyone has had bad things happen to them. If you hold on to it, you're perpetuating the damage, and there's no wisdom in that. It doesn't matter what terrible loss or injury happened to you. I would never want to minimize what happened. But one thing I know for sure. Whatever happened is in the past. You can't change the past. No one can change the past. If your foot was blown off by a land mine, if you were raped, if you lost all your money, if you lost your family in an accident—yes, these were terrible things, but by holding on to that memory and keeping it fresh you join in perpetuating the damage with whatever or whoever did that to you. It's a form of double victimization. First you're victimized by whatever bad thing happened to you. Then you victimize yourself by keeping it alive within yourself.

"I can't help it," you might say. I understand. But have you really tried?

Have you tried not talking about it? Beyond a certain point, all talking does is keep the wound raw and prevent it from healing.

Have you tried not thinking about it? To do that takes a little bit of discipline. Every time the memory of your loss or your guilt or your regret comes into your mind, immediately try to think about something else. If your memory of loss never feels welcome in your mind, it will gradually get discouraged and slink away. This may take a little time, but it will happen. And it will turn loss into enormous growth, because you'll have taken yourself out of the victim role.

Most of all, have you tried embracing life? Have you put your energy into thinking about all the wonderful parts of your life you've stayed away from and finding ways to throw yourself into new relationships, new activities?

Remember, if you don't move on, you're adding damage to damage.

You *will* let go at some point, you know. Most people do eventually. You will get to the point where you say, "I don't know why I held on and obsessed over that loss for so long." If you're going to let go eventually, why not let go now?

The other fork in the road is going into therapy. If you've had trouble letting go, there's something you're getting from holding on. Maybe you're getting off on everyone feeling sorry for you. Maybe you're giving yourself a way out of having to do something with your life. You may need a therapist to help you see what holding on to loss does for you. The key is finding a therapist who will help you find a way to turn away from your loss and start embracing your life. If you're at this point, admit you need help and get it.

Every ounce of emotional energy that's tied up with loss makes you old and tired inside and prevents you from getting the wonderful benefits that come from putting your emotional energy into the wonderful things life has to offer.

10

Envy Is Poison

Emotional Energy Booster #10

You're on a small boat in the middle of a big sea, and the sea is rolling. There you are standing on deck and you go up and you go down and up and down and then you tilt to starboard and then you tilt to port and then up and down again. Soon you're gripped by seasickness and you turn green.

There's another part of our lives where we talk about turning green—envy—and it's really for very much the same reason. Instead of having solid ground under your feet, instead of feeling strong and balanced and secure, you've been gripped by nauseating, powerful forces you can't control. You've been carried away by a merciless unreasoning sea of envy.

And just the way seasickness destroys physical energy, when people are gripped by envy their emotional energy is utterly wiped out. Whatever hope and focus they might have had, envy comes along, scoops them up, hollows out their stomach, and makes them weak and sick inside.

Why is this, and what can we do about it?

How Envy Makes You
Emotionally Exhausted

There was a mystery about Mike. It's true he was under a lot of pressure and he had a lot of frustration to deal with, but his utter emotional exhaustion seemed to be disproportionate. There had to be an explanation somewhere. And there was.

Mike, 42: "I'll admit that I have a lot on my plate. Things are crazy with my little business—just the usual hassles and pressures, nothing big, but it's constant. Of course, now I'm engaged and we're trying to find a new place to live. There's a lot happening, but it's just everyday life. The problem is that I feel overwhelmed. I could never admit this to anyone, but most days I feel like staying in bed with the covers pulled over my head. I want to say no to everything. I know I should be able to handle all this, but it's like there's something broken inside me and I feel completely overwhelmed.

"What happened? How did I get the rug pulled out from under me?"

I'd just met Mike. I didn't know the answer to his questions. You always have to tease these things out. But sometimes the best way to find an answer is to try to figure out *when* a person first started feeling a certain way and then look at what was actually going on in their lives at that exact time.

And that's what I pushed Mike to do. It turned out he'd been feeling pretty good about himself a few years ago, even though things in his life weren't any easier. Then Mike said, "You know, it's funny. I started feeling really low around the time I went to my twentieth high school reunion."

"Really?" I said. "What happened there?"

It turned out that at the reunion Mike ran into the guys who'd been his best buddies on the football team. These were guys who'd been Mike's equals, no better on the football field than he was, no smarter off the field than he was. Now, twenty years later, they each had something that made Mike feel like a goofball who'd been doing nothing but waste time.

Mike: "I had a sinking feeling after I talked to those guys. We were catching up, but every detail went through me like a hot knife. It was everything. One of the guys had a Porsche, and I'm a million years away from buying a Porsche. They were all married with kids, and my fiancée and I are still not sure about each other after five years. One was working on Wall Street, making tons of money. Another had built up a chain of pizza shops that was very successful. On the drive home my fiancée commented on how quiet I was. It was like the stuffing had been knocked out of me.

"You know what it was like? It's like you're running a race and you see all these guys ahead of you and they're better runners anyway. What's the point? Why not quit?"

It's surprising how often envy attacks us. A person's going along in life. He hears about someone who has something he doesn't have. He talks to someone who can do something he can't do. Maybe he just sees someone who *looks* like he has the money or the family or the happy marriage he doesn't have. And it's like a debilitating poison has entered his system. There's a sour, curdling sensation in the pit of his being. Often he feels a surge of anger, but the anger rots into a state of regret and helplessness.

Diagnostic Question #10

Do you feel one down compared to others? Do you have a sense of missing out in your life? Would you say that you frequently compare yourself to others and feel resentful?

A **yes** *answer to any of these questions means that this secret will give you a big boost of emotional energy.*

If envy were a chemical, the Environmental Protection Agency would outlaw it. It's that toxic. Show me a person with emotional problems and I'll show you someone wrestling with envy. For example, they've done studies of the impact of unemployment on mental health. Back in the 1930s, when millions were unemployed, people were less depressed about being out of work. Why? Because there was a sense that everyone was in the same boat. Everyone was struggling. But in the sixties and eighties, when there were brief periods of high unemployment, people suffered more psychological pain. Why? Because they were envious of all the other people who had good jobs.

One of the worst parts of envy, and one of the reasons it can be so deadly to our emotional energy, is the way it ambushes us. We're going along just fine, and suddenly we're talking to a friend over lunch and she makes some comment that flattens us. Let's say she talks about how when she got sick her boyfriend took such good care of her. That's not such a big deal. But when we got sick, the important person in our lives didn't take such good care of us. Instant envy. Instant emotional exhaustion.

So I'll put it to you. If you're not feeling as energetic as you'd like, there's probably someone you're envying, and this is draining you.

Sunlight Kills Envy

Nothing looks more pathetic than envy when it's seen for what it is. And that makes envy relatively straightforward to get rid of.

Scott looked like a happy, healthy guy. He looked like the golf pro that he was. A regular on the PGA tour. But he wasn't always so glowing.

Scott, 33: "I don't think there's a golf pro out there who hasn't had nightmares about Tiger Woods. This is a tough enough game by itself, and the competition is fierce, but then this guy comes along and he's the eight-hundred-pound gorilla, and the rest of us are midgets. He gets all the attention, makes all the money, has all the fun. We fight over crumbs.

"At least that's the sick way a lot of guys think. They haven't recovered from the Tiger factor. It's like as long as he's there, they're doomed.

"I felt the same way. It took me a long time to get on the tour, and I don't feel my hold on it is secure. At first Tiger made me feel like a damned fool. What was the point? I'd never be his equal. And even if I won a major, I'd never get the attention he gets. I wanted to pack it in.

"So early one morning I'm out there taking a practice round. It's the ninth hole, par four, a tricky dogleg. But there's dew on the grass, everything smells great, and the sun is raking across the fairway. Every blade of grass has its own little shadow. And I tee off and hit this sweet drive, nice length, right where I wanted it to go. Just a nice little shot.

"And I realized how much I loved this. Why should anyone, even Tiger, have the power to spoil it for me? In fact, no one did have the power to spoil it. Even if I were playing with Tiger in a twosome and he were beating me at every hole, how could that spoil the sun and the way everything smelled and the joy of hitting a ball? What does one thing have to do with another? How does what someone else has take away from what I have?"

Scott had found the key. Envy is a weird force. It's so powerful when you're caught in its grip. And yet it collapses like a house of cards when you expose it to the cold light of day.

Before envy strikes, you are you, with all the pluses and minuses in your life. Envy grabs you and pulls you in directions that have nothing to do with where you were. Ultimately it sucks you into a game you can't win. Let's face it. The world is filled with people who have things we don't have. There's always someone smarter, richer, thinner, better-looking, with better stuff. And you're going to run into these people when you least need it.

How to Envy-Proof Yourself

This is what high-energy people do to pluck out the thorn of envy.

• *Be aware of all the ways you're pricked by envy.* Note how you see someone on TV or read about someone in a magazine and suddenly you feel mysteriously cast down. Think about the people in your family who stir up your envy juices. Notice how you chat with someone at work and they make some little comment about something they have and suddenly you're bummed out. Follow the feeling. That's the impact of envy on you.

We're vulnerable to envy when we've experienced a loss or failure. Your dog just died and the teacher just told you your kid is stupid. That's bad enough. Then you see someone walking their dog and someone else tells you how bright their kid is. Boom! The demons of envy attack you.

But we don't like to think of ourselves as envious. We often don't feel envy directly. What we experience is hearing about someone and feeling depressed. I remember for years feeling depressed on Sunday mornings. That's bizarre. Who ever heard of Sunday morning depression? But every Sunday morning I'd read the papers. They were filled with articles about people going places and doing things. I was just getting started, and I felt invisible. There were all these people who had what I didn't have in spite of how hard I worked. I felt depressed, but it was really envy. When you realize how these land mines of envy explode under your feet, they lose their power.

• *Know that envy is bad for your health.* You're already motivated by what you want for yourself. All envy does is make you feel frustrated. All envy does is take you outside yourself. All it does is remind you of what you don't have and force you to play a game you can't possibly win, since there will always be people who have what's beyond your reach.

• *Realize that envy is mostly an exercise in ignorance.* You know how messy and complicated your life is from the inside. That person you're envying—all you know about his life is from the outside. You don't know about his frustrations. You don't know about his pain. You don't know about the disasters he's standing on the precipice of. The chances are you're envying someone whose life you wouldn't want if you got it.

• *Focus on how much better you'll feel without envy.* Suppose you didn't get knocked out by every little thing someone has that you don't. Then you'd be happy and hopeful. Well, why not start anticipating that now? Specifically, look forward to feeling good about yourself and your life because no one and nothing will have the power to make you feel bad.

• *Count your blessings.* We've heard this so many times we forget how important it is. It's an enormously powerful entrée to more emotional energy. It is what high-energy people do. Look at what you have in and of itself. Make yourself aware of all the positive things in your life. And actively feel grateful for them, without comparing yourself to anyone else.

Emotional energy booster #10
In the land of emotional energy, green means danger.
Never envy anyone.

Sometimes you have to go through a personal crisis to get to the point where you can enjoy what you've got. That's what happened to Cheryl.

Cheryl, 32: "The story about blind people is that we're content because we've never known anything else. But it's not true. Yeah, I was happy as a little kid. Kids accept whatever their lives are. But at thirteen it got to me. I wanted to go to parties and be normal. And it hit me how I'll never be normal. I went to a regular high school, and I was envious of every girl there. I wanted to be pretty. I asked my mom if I was pretty, and she said yes, I was very pretty. But she was my mom. How would I ever know?

"I think I was in a funk all through high school, through my sophomore year in college. I'm on the outside looking in, except I can't look in.

"Then I started getting to know this boy, and he seemed interested in me. And I liked him too. But I'm suspicious. What kind of guy wants a blind girl? So I guess I was kind of cold toward him. But he hung in there and took me out a few times. We had a good time when I remembered to relax. Finally I asked him why he wanted to be with a blind girl. And he said, and I remember his words, 'I don't want to be with a blind girl. I want to be with you.' It's funny. He just liked me. I asked him if he thought I was pretty. He surprised me. He was so honest. He said, 'I'll tell you this. You're prettier than average. You've got a great smile. And a great figure. And beautiful black hair. You're a lot prettier for a girl than I am for a boy.'

"That seemed so honest. He could've said anything. How would I have known? So I believed him. Then it hit me. College was half over, and this is when you're supposed to have a good time. Enjoy what you can while you can. I'd always be blind. Nothing could ever change that. So I could suffer because I didn't have someone else's life or I could enjoy my own."

Cheryl was smarter at nineteen than most of us are at any age. She accepted where she was starting from and what she had. She knew that the comparison game was a loser's game. When you fall victim to envy, you'll always lose, not because you're really disadvantaged but because emotionally you're in a disadvantaged place. Cheryl understood that she'd be compounding the disadvantage of her blindness with a far more emotionally destructive disadvantage if she stopped herself from enjoying her life as it was.

Envy is terrible because it stops you from seeing who you really are and what you already have.

11

Guilt Is Stupid

Emotional Energy Booster #11

One of the most interesting and dramatic secrets of people who are super-charged with emotional energy is that they're not carrying around a sense of guilt about anything. Sure, they may feel bad that they did something or other in the past, but it doesn't weigh on them.

That's the point. They get energy by resolving their guilt.

How Guilt Weighs You Down

Make no mistake about it. Guilt is a terrible burden. Few people know that better than Barbara. But I also learned from her that no matter what kind of guilt we're carrying around, there is a way to let go of the burden. And when you do, you'll feel like a whole new you.

Barbara, 29: "I'm feeling good about myself and my life for the first time ever now. It's amazing. You don't know what you're missing when you're carrying guilt around. It's like someone who's been deaf from birth—you know there are people who hear sounds, but you have no idea what that means unless somehow by some miracle you start hearing sounds yourself.

"I guess I had a kind of miracle in my life. I almost didn't make it. The low point came the night I was arrested for drunk driving. It was the day after I got fired from the band where I was the lead singer. We were starting to be famous, and then almost overnight I was practically homeless and broke. How did I spin out of control like that? It all came from terrible guilt.

"I can't remember ever not feeling guilty. And there's a reason for that. I was five and my eight-year-old brother Eddie and I were in the country for the summer. Upstate New York. It was the real country, and we'd spend part of the day roaming around and never see another person. We found this swimming hole. Maybe it was part of an old quarry, I don't know. But there was this high rock, I mean really high, and my brother and I were standing at the edge of it looking down at the dark water. And like the little brat that I was, I kept saying, 'Jump, jump, jump.' I wanted to see him jump into the water below and make a big splash.

"He obviously was scared to do it. But when your bratty little sister dares you . . . anyway, he jumped. I watched him go into the water, and he didn't come out. It turned out that there were rocks below the surface of the water, and he hit his head and drowned.

"I ran to our cottage and told my mother that Eddie had jumped in the water and disappeared. I never told anyone that I'd made him jump. But the grown-ups asked me so many questions about where he was when he jumped and why he jumped that they made me feel even guiltier for not having stopped him. I just thought, 'Wow, if they only knew that I basically pushed him in.'

"So there I am growing up thinking I'd killed my brother, whom I loved and worshiped. He'd been my hero.

"There was nothing I could do about my guilt. It's like being a hunchback or something. It was a fact I carried around inside me: I was an evil, horrible, destructive person, so much so that if the knowledge of it got out, it would destroy everything around me. You want guilt? That's guilt.

"So I'm going along living with that guilt, and in my last year at Berklee, ready to launch my music career, I get pregnant. Immediately—because of my brother, of course—I'm thinking there's no way I'm going to get an abortion. I'm not against it in principle, but I personally am not entitled to it. So I'm thinking I'm going to have a baby. I think I can deal with it. But about a month before I ended up giving birth I just knew there was no way I could be a mother at that point. Obviously I was nowhere in my life, and I was very, very unhappy. I'd been paying a big price for my guilt over my brother. I was always tired, always having trouble concentrating. I did have a great singing voice. Without that I think I'd have been a bum.

"I gave my daughter up for adoption three days after she was born. I knew then and I know now that it was the right thing to do. But still, I had a whole new load of guilt from that. A mother just doesn't give her kid away. It's a terrible thing to do.

"So now I'm thinking I'm a total monster. Okay, but I joined a couple of bands and started to get known. And I feel terribly guilty about *that*. Right away I see that I'm having a very lucky career. I know I don't deserve it. I deserve punishment, not reward.

"That's when I started to self-destruct. It's not that I wanted to destroy myself. It's that I just couldn't go on. Showing up for gigs, getting up in the morning, getting dressed . . . everything was too hard. Drinking was great—it didn't make anything easier, but it helped me not see how hard everything was.

"After my arrest and after I was thrown out of the band and I had nothing and nowhere to go, I called up my old singing teacher—she was my mentor—and by a kind of miracle she offered to take me in for a while. For a time I didn't talk to her; I didn't do anything. I just sat around her house, numb. Eventually Alice told me I could either start talking or get the hell out. I started talking.

"All the stuff about all my guilt came out. Alice wasn't a therapist, but she was a singing teacher and had the approach that for every problem there's some little technical adjustment you can make to solve it. I always tell people now if you need a therapist, go to a singing teacher.

"Also, I'd never talked to anyone about any of this before. Guilt does that to you. It locks you up alone with your problem.

"Anyway, Alice kind of led me through a kind of cleansing process. It was just a Q-and-A. With my brother, for example, she asked me if you can hold a five-year-old responsible for anything she does. Particularly when she's just acting like a normal five-year-old. Then she put it to me. If you excessively, inappropriately punish a normal little kid for doing what any little kid would do, isn't that a far worse crime? She said, 'If you want to feel guilty, feel guilty about feeling guilty. And then just stop, because you didn't do anything that any other little kid wouldn't do.'

"As for giving my child up for adoption, she asked me what I'd done that was really so bad. 'After all,' she said, 'you gave your kid a chance at a much better family to grow up in.' Where was the damage? Why feel guilty when you made things better, not worse?

"And as for my being lucky as a singer, she said it was just nuts to feel guilty over that. Had I stolen anything from anyone? Of course not. That's how things worked. Different people are born with different gifts. 'But,' she said, 'there's one thing and *only* one thing you do when you get a gift. You act grateful. You put the gift in a place of honor. And you try to find a way to somehow return the favor.' She said she wished she had my gift and my luck. But all she wants of me is that I use it to the fullest and then do things to help others.

"'I'll make it real simple,' she said. 'Life is about making good things happen. If feeling guilty isn't going to make anything good happen—and obviously it isn't—then just stop it.'

"I took in everything Alice said. It made my head spin. I'd been such a fool. But I didn't know exactly what to do next. So I asked her. What she then said was amazing. 'Look,' she said, 'you've got two choices. And only two. If you're actually responsible for hurting someone, then you've got to do something so big and meaningful that you make it clear to yourself that you're paying the price for what you did. Or you've got to let it go. But your suffering this way—no one benefits. Fix it or forget it. If you can't do one or the other, then you're just full of crap.'

"It's funny. It was hard to feel guilty for my brother dying when I actually thought about treating it like a real crime. And if I wouldn't put myself in jail, why not let myself out of jail? And it was the same about putting my daughter up for adoption."

Ending the Guilt

Barbara had an enormous surge of energy once she decided to either pay for her crimes or let go of her guilt. She started searching out singing jobs. She began writing songs. Her voiced opened up. She grew confident. Perhaps most surprising, she started feeling a surge of sensuality flowing through her veins. It made her realize that part of her had felt dead inside for a very long time. But that part of her hadn't been dead. It had just been exhausted from the burden of guilt she'd been carrying around.

I've learned that you can't help anyone get rid of guilt unless they want to get rid of it. As crazy as it sounds, some people just *like* feeling guilty. It makes them feel important without actually having to do anything important. It makes them feel alive without having to participate in life. It's a way to quit, and so it's perfect for quitters. Let's face it, there are people who don't want more emotional energy. Their view is that it's better to live a small life with little energy than a big life with a lot of energy.

But if you're a real energy seeker, you have to look at the issue of guilt in your life.

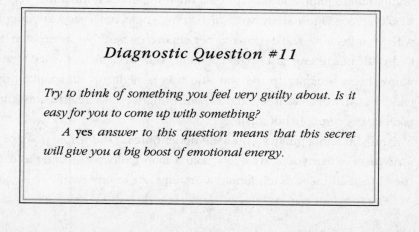

Diagnostic Question #11

Try to think of something you feel very guilty about. Is it easy for you to come up with something?

A **yes** *answer to this question means that this secret will give you a big boost of emotional energy.*

If you feel it's a sad waste to sit around feeling guilty and if you welcome the thought of having more emotional energy, the way out of guilt
requires you to face it honestly so you can put it behind you.

What you're going to do is basically put yourself on trial. Right here.
Right now. At the end of the process you'll have clarity and, one way or
another, an end to your feeling of guilt.

First step. Did you actually commit a crime, not necessarily in the strict
legal sense but in the human sense? After all, there's no need to proceed
to sentencing if you can't be held responsible for committing any crime.
Barbara committed no crime whatsoever when she put her child up for
adoption. At that point she had no means to bring her baby up properly,
but she was able to give her to a wonderful family. Where's the crime
when you're making things better?

Then ask yourself if you were really responsible. You're certainly not
responsible if you didn't do anything wrong.

Lots of people feel guilty because bad things happened to people they
care about. Maybe they failed to prevent the bad thing from happening.
But they probably couldn't have prevented it. For example, if you're in a
relationship with someone who messes up his life, why should you feel
guilty unless you put a gun to his head and made him mess up his life?

And you're not responsible if you were doing the best you could for a
person of your age and background. Barbara wasn't responsible for her
brother's accidental death because she was only five years old, and by
urging him to jump she wasn't doing anything that a normal five-year-old
wouldn't do. One elderly woman I know spent her last years crippled
with guilt because she'd spanked her children when they were little. She
hadn't beaten them, just spanked them. But women of her generation
who'd been brought up the way she was brought up *all* spanked their
children. At worst what she did is something we now realize was a mistake. It was certainly not a crime.

And you're not guilty if you were under duress. The whole point of *Les
Misérables* is that you can't really hold a man guilty for stealing a loaf of
bread to feed his starving family. Certainly not in any moral sense. And

lots of the seemingly bad things we've done were under the duress of desperation, panic, raging hormones, and many other forces.

And it's not a crime at all if nothing all that bad really happened. Did someone really suffer as a result of what you did? You broke up with someone. The other person was hurt. But come on, people get dumped all the time. And people recover.

Maybe the person you dumped went into a tailspin. But remember, it's not a crime if you're not really responsible, and you can't possibly be responsible for whether someone holds himself together in the face of an emotional shock. And it's not a crime if all you did is be who you are. Did you even do anything at all? You got emotional. People around you got upset at that. Tough noogies. That's who you are.

And it's not a crime if all you did was a perfectly normal thing that people typically do in those situations. Does that apply to you? You goofed off in college, let's say. That's a shame, but you were twenty years old, for goodness' sake. People that age do that.

All right, then—if you didn't commit a crime, then the trial must be brought to a halt. The charges must be dismissed. It's *over*. Now you *have* to stop feeling guilty.

Well? Still feel guilty? Then you must find the crime you think you committed and move on to the second step.

Second step. If you did something that amounts to a real crime, you have to stand up and plead guilty. You know the truth. You know if you actually did something you shouldn't have done that actually hurt someone.

If so, now the trial proceeds to the penalty phase. Now you have to do something meaningful to compensate for that crime.

If you specifically hurt another person, repay that person. If that person can't be repaid, repay your debt to society or to someone else. Do something real that will discharge that guilt. Set up a program for yourself. A lifetime sentence if necessary, if you're really responsible for a crime that was serious. By a "sentence" I mean something specific, such as doing volunteer work every Saturday for a long period of time. Or giving a significant amount of money to a person or a cause. The point is that you can't cheat. Your "sentence" can't be so small that it doesn't make a dent in your guilt. But it can't be open-ended either. You've got to be able to say, "When I've done *that,* then I'll have paid for my deed." The miracle is that even if you give yourself a life sentence, the emotional burden of guilt is over once you *start* serving the sentence.

Emotional energy booster #11
If paying for your crime doesn't make sense, let your guilt go—
why feel guilty if there's nothing to pay for? If you really are
responsible for doing something bad, then you've got to pay for
it—but why feel guilty if you're paying for what you did?
Either way the burden of guilt will drop away.

The boost in emotional energy that comes with either letting go of guilt or starting to pay for your "crime" can be described only by people who've done this. It's too dramatic, too deep, for anyone to believe unless you've lived through it. Some people describe it as feeling like suddenly being able to see when you hadn't even realized you were blind. Some people describe it as like going to sleep weighing eight hundred pounds and waking up perfectly fit at your ideal weight.

You can feel again, have hope, enjoy life. That's emotional energy.

Special Issue:

Emotional Energy and
Health Problems

Remember the basic energy equation:

Complete energy = physical energy + emotional energy

The good news about emotional energy is that when your body gives you trouble and you have less physical energy, emotional energy can come to the rescue and compensate for what's missing. That way, overall, you can maintain your total energy.

Unfortunately, the bad news about physical problems is that sometimes they can sap your emotional energy. So it becomes very important when you get sick or you're trying to recover from an injury that you recognize the ways you're becoming emotionally exhausted and that you use the secrets in this book to maintain and build up your emotional energy.

I've talked to many people who have dealt with a difficult medical condition, and here are some suggestions they say work best for maintaining emotional energy.

• *Recognize that physical problems have emotional consequences.* When I get a cold, I get blue. I used to psychoanalyze this, but I now know that it's the way energy works. Lowered physical energy lowers your emotional energy. Stress, discouragement, low self-esteem, fear, anger, and other negative emotional responses may very well sap your emotional energy. It doesn't mean there's anything wrong with you. It does mean that you have to do things to deal with it. You can't be in denial. Fortunately you're holding in your hand a book full of specific things to do that will not only lift up your depleted emotional energy but will make it possible for you to actually compensate for your lowered physical energy. But you have to do them. The minute you're hit by a medical or physical problem, use one of the secrets in this book to increase your emotional energy.

• *Sleep.* Nothing has more powerful healing properties than sleep. You have to make it a priority. You can't be brave or try to tough it out. Think of sleep as the special repair shop that allows physical and emotional energy to heal. If you've not been getting enough, this is the time to get it. If you have been getting enough, this is the time to get more. Sleep may not sound like a big deal, but if you went to a support group for people going through what you're going through, you'd hear how important sleep is.

• *Become fully informed about your physical condition.* Sometimes when we're scared we don't want to know about what we're going through. We're afraid it will make us more scared. But people who feel they're on top of what they're going through, people who feel hopeful, smart, and effective, have always worked the hardest to learn the most about their condition. Ask someone who's been battling cancer. Darkness is despair. Light is hope. Knowledge is power.

• *Don't let your condition define you.* We've all heard about those old people in Florida who sit around on benches talking about nothing but their aches and pains. We're all turned off by that, whatever our age. And we're right to be turned off. It's one thing to deal with a health problem. It's another to let yourself be dragged down by it. Here's what people report works. Don't talk about your condition all the time. Don't let it stop you from doing what you need to do. Define what business as usual means for you and then keep on with it. Your physical problem is not your life. Make sure you have your life.

• *Get support.* This suggestion goes hand in hand with the previous one. If most of the time you're not going to pay attention to your physical condition or even allow other people to question you about it—because you're trying to forget it—some of the time you're going to need a place where you can talk about it with people who understand. This could be a once-a-week support group. It could be a friend who once dealt with what you're dealing with now. It could be a very sympathetic person you chat with from time to time. But you need to have this support precisely so that the rest of the time you can pay attention to your life and not your problem.

• *Have appropriate expectations for yourself.* It might be that you need to expect yourself to do work of a different quality, or to do a different kind of work. Or it might simply be that you give yourself the gift of changing your expectations of yourself so they fit your current circumstances. The point is to accept the fact that you need to feel good about yourself for doing things differently from the way you've been doing them.

• *Don't let anyone push you beyond your limits.* When you're dealing with a physical challenge, particularly if this is something new, the people in your life really don't know how difficult things are for you. Plus they may be a little scared or threatened. So they may continue to ask you to do things that you could once do but you can no longer do. And you won't want to disappoint them. So you'll try to live up to their expectations, and either you'll fail or you'll burn yourself out. And then your emotional energy will be in far worse shape than it would've been otherwise. Save yourself from that. Say no, and say no a lot. Say no more than you really need to. The worst that'll happen is that you'll find yourself with excess energy.

• *Find ways to take more control of your life.* The psychological impact of physical problems comes from your body taking control of you. It's like you've been kidnapped. This is emotionally painful. The only solution is to take back some control. And the only way to take back control is to make decisions, big and little. Decide that you're going to buy a new couch. Decide that you're going to deal with your physical pain the way you want to deal with it. Decide that you are going to stop talking to someone in your life who's a bummer. Decide that you're going to make a change in the kind of help you're getting. Decide to cut your hair. Every little thing you decide to do to take some control will rebuild your emotional energy.

• *Look for improvements*. No matter what you're dealing with physically, you can be aware of changes that are happening for the better. Notice how your pain is diminished. Notice how your symptoms are coming a little less frequently. Notice how you're getting a little better managing your symptoms. Notice how you're getting better at accepting your condition. Notice how you're getting better at asking for help. No matter what, there can and will be improvements somewhere, and you need to focus on that instead of on the problem.

• *Find the hope*. There's hope somewhere. That bad cold that seems to have gone on forever? Bad colds always finally come to an end. The chronic pain you're in as a result of a bad car crash? New therapies and the cumulative impact of everything you're doing will finally cause your pain to go away. A mysterious disease? Somewhere, someone has seen this condition before, knows what it is, and knows how to deal with it. And there's probably a group for it too. Even when you learn there's something seriously wrong with you, you can get the hope that comes from feeling that finally your problem's been figured out and now you can begin to solve it. Every health problem means facing some temporary or permanent loss. That's a fact, even if it's just a cold. But once you accept your necessary loss as a given, there are endless ways to find new hope. Look for it. Embrace it. It's real. And your hope will give you emotional energy.

12

Keep Your Flywheel Spinning

Emotional Energy Booster #12

People talk about finding your life's passion, and that's great, but from the point of view of emotional energy maybe it's just a little too grandiose for most of us. Anything that's hard to find, hard to balance with the rest of your life, can be more intimidating and draining than energizing.

So I talk about keeping your flywheel spinning. All that means is that there's something you're interested in, that you care about, that gives you emotional energy. That's your flywheel, and everyone can benefit from having one. I got the term from a mechanical device—often it's a big, heavy spinning disk like in your car's transmission—that stores energy and then gives it back to you when you need it. When I was a kid my favorite thing in the playground was the little merry-go-round the kids would push until it was going as fast as it could, and then we'd all jump on. That merry-go-round was a flywheel. Because it was so heavy and big, it took a while to get going, but once it got going, it would keep on going. We'd laugh and laugh. It was so much fun.

We all need a flywheel. If you're a high-energy person, you definitely have one: something you're passionately interested in. It's always present in your life. Whatever else is happening, when you connect with your interest, and do something about it, it gives you energy. It doesn't matter what it is. It might be something that seems stupid to others. But if you're getting energy from it, what's stupid about that? It's having the love that counts, not what the love is for.

Leslie, 29: "I know a lot of people love to collect antiques. What I love to do is to collect antique *recipes*. That's right. It's pretty involved. I browse through secondhand bookstores looking for very old cookbooks. I try to dig up nineteenth-century letters where sometimes someone will write down a recipe. There are lots of places to look. It's a lot of fun, but that's really just where the fun begins. The thing is that the ingredients are often unobtainable now or they're very different. The measurements are sometimes not mentioned at all. So you have to keep experimenting many times to finally cook up a dish that is both authentic and actually tastes good.

"My poor husband. First of all, I have to throw away a lot of dishes that don't come out right. But I just say that it's a sacrifice on the altar of art. I've got to be honest with you. Old-fashioned cooking, from the eighteenth and nineteenth centuries back to Queen Elizabeth and Henry the Eighth and even Eleanor of Aquitaine, isn't always to modern tastes, any more than you'd want to wear the clothes they wore back then. They really did cook up pheasant's tongues—and it's marvelous—but it's not what our Burger King generation wants to eat.

"I feel like I'm re-creating history. When I make some dish from a very old recipe, I might be eating something that no one has eaten for hundreds of years. It's the closest you can get to living for just a moment inside the skin of someone who lived long ago.

"All I can say is that for me it's so exciting, so thrilling, so special. I feel like one of those archaeologists who find a dinosaur bone no one's seen before, except that for me it's like I find the bone and then bring the dinosaur back to life. And of course there are other people like me. And we're always exchanging recipes and ideas. I'm doing something that's so much fun and yet something that feels so important in its own little way. It just feels wonderful. I always have something to look forward to."

There you have it. In this story you heard all the ingredients for this emotional energy booster. Something fun, involving, absorbing. Something special. Something that fills your life with adventures to look forward to. Something that's connected with who you are or what you care about.

Diagnostic Question #12

Is there something in your life you're really interested in, and are you pursuing it?

*A **no** answer to this question means that this secret will give you a big boost of emotional energy.*

Your Own Private Shortcut
to Emotional Energy

Maybe many others share what it is you love. Maybe yours is a solitary passion. But the key is the sense that *it* gives *you* energy, not the other way around. It's not something you have to make yourself do. There's no procrastination or feeling of being blocked. It gives you emotional energy to think about it, it gives you energy while you're involved with it, and it leaves you with energy when you have to stop. Just anticipating the next time you're going to hook up with it gets you up in the morning and gets you through an otherwise unrewarding day.

Robert, 32: "I'm a high school math teacher, and I like teaching, and I really like the kids. But I teach because it lets me indulge in my real passion, which you can't do with most jobs because you don't get the time off.

"Maybe I'm even nuts about this, but what I really, really love is going somewhere very far away, very exotic, with my bicycle and just bicycling through places that maybe haven't been seen ever before by the eyes of someone on a bicycle. At least they're far away and the fact that I'm pedaling through means I can see details that you don't see when you're driving. It's easy for me to stop at places no one stops at.

"I've cycled on dirt paths in the Amazon jungle. I've cycled through the foothills of Nepal. I've cycled around the tip of South America one winter (it's summer down there) during school vacation. I've cycled along back roads in Mississippi, Alabama, and Louisiana. I've even cycled through the Greek Islands retracing the path Odysseus took. Thank God I have the kind of mind where I remember what I see. It's like I'm making a movie while I'm pedaling along; I can close my eyes and see these movies.

"I always want to go somewhere special. My next idea is to bicycle to Timbuktu. You know that it used to be a very important trading town. They say it's not much now, but I say, hey, it's Timbuktu. It's also very far away from anything and you're almost in the Sahara Desert, so this is going to be tough to pull off. But that's part of what I like, spending weeks and months investigating whether something like this is really possible and then planning for how I'm going to do it.

"There are so many different reasons people travel. I think of what I love to do as a way of being intimate with the world. It feels very special."

Leslie and Robert may be bad examples because they're unusual. Millions of people get just as big an energy boost from abandoning themselves to a garden-variety interest such as golf or needlework. It doesn't matter how special it is to anyone else. What matters is how special it is to you.

So what do you love to do?

Finding Your Own Private Shortcut

Maybe you already have something. It could be exercising every chance you get. It could be your work or taking care of your family. Whatever it is, make sure you realize what a great source of emotional energy this is for you.

Maybe there are things in your life you're interested in and enjoy, but you haven't been doing much with them recently. Well, you should. If it's something you really care about that gives you energy, you ought to make it a big deal in your life. It's not an indulgence. It's a necessity.

Or maybe it's hard for you to point to anything and say, "That's what I love." Well, there are so many ways to get emotional energy, it's not the end of the world if you don't find something right away. But look for it. Just keep an eye open. Pay attention to what you respond to positively and with interest. Prepare to surprise yourself. For lots of us the things that turn out to be what we truly love were interests we never could've predicted.

Remember: If you're open, you will find things you're truly interested in. We all need this emotionally. You can have a crappy day at work. Your relationship can fall into a bad place. Someone you love can move far away. All of these are depressing, discouraging events, things that make us want to go to bed and pull the covers over our heads. This is a reality in everyone's life. But think about what this means. It means that your emotional energy is a hostage to events you can't control. You get emotional energy when everything goes right. But you lose it when things go wrong.

It's terrible to live that way. You need something that generates a steady hum of emotional energy no matter what's going on, so that you can always turn to it and start feeling good again. If you find something you love, the flywheel effect will always be there to give you emotional energy. When Leslie and Robert have bad days, they still have something they love and look forward to that puts it all in perspective.

In the worst of times, having a flywheel can save you from going down the tubes emotionally.

Judy, 38: "My husband died last year, and I wanted to die too. We'd been married for seventeen years. He was the only man I'd ever loved. And, you know, marriages have ups and downs, but we were always best friends and lovers no matter what. When Larry died, I knew I'd be alone for the rest of my life because there'd never be anyone to replace him.

"My sons were sixteen and fourteen when their father died. I know you say you keep going for the kids' sake, and you do, but they already had lives of their own and they're going off to college soon enough. All the children in the world can't make up for the loss of a husband like mine.

"So what kept me going? I didn't have to work. Larry had life insurance. I'd get up in the morning to see the kids off to school. And then I'd go back to bed and stay there. Just before they were due home I'd crawl out, fix myself up so I wouldn't look like I'd spent all day in bed, and then do whatever had to be done. My life was empty, and I was empty.

"I was in mourning, but I was afraid of what would happen when I stopped because I knew there was nothing else. When I'd stop feeling sad, I'd stop feeling anything, and that's when I was afraid I'd kill myself.

"Let me tell you what saved my life. You should know that Larry's parents had been refugees from Hitler, and Larry and I had gotten active in some refugee organizations. It started at our temple, but then we branched out, because, let's face it, there aren't many Jewish refugees in America these days. And I've always thought a refugee was a refugee.

"So we'd been involved in advocacy and outreach and direct services. I'd been very busy with this. You're talking about people who have nothing, and they're lost in a strange country where they don't speak the language and they don't know the customs. I don't know why I'd gotten so caught up in it. You'd have to go back a long time in my own family before you found any refugees. I think I just felt that these were people where you could really do something to help their lives. I'm a very practical person. I just really cared.

"I don't remember now how many weeks it was after Larry died, but I was still a completely broken woman. Then I got a call from a woman at our temple. She offers me her condolences, but then she starts telling me about this refugee family from Indonesia, where they had all these problems, and there're about twelve people in this family and they need all kinds of help. I'm the only one available. It's an emergency. It's always an emergency.

"With every fiber of my being I wanted to say 'No, I don't care; I'm not interested.' I resented having to get out of bed. And I was about to say no, but what somehow got to me was the thought that this is what I do. I do this. I help refugees. *It's who I am.* Larry's death left me with nothing. But if I say no to his, I'm leaving *myself* with nothing.

"It almost physically hurt to leave the little womb of pain I'd built for myself. But you can't think about yourself when you show up in some little crappy two-room apartment with twelve people in it and they don't know how to buy food and they don't know how to use appliances or anything. I have a gift for communicating with people where none of us speaks the same language. I roll up my sleeves and I dig in.

"A few hours later I realized that this was my passion. It had always been my passion. No one could save me from what had happened to me, but I could save these people from the terrible place they were in right now. And after them there was a world of refugees out there.

"It was like I'd flipped a switch. One minute I can't get out of bed. The next minute I'm swept away by something I care about. I stopped thinking about myself, but I did realize that I felt happy and alive again. It was like I'd been unplugged from life, and then I found these people and then I got plugged in again. Suddenly I had all the energy in the world."

Emotional energy booster #12
Find something you're truly interested in
that you can always turn to.

A flywheel is there to save you whenever your energy runs low. One day it might save your life.

13

If You Don't Get Help, You're Doing It Wrong

Emotional Energy Booster #13

A friend of mine found herself having to deal with ovarian cancer. That's a scary condition for anyone. Death is a possibility. Treatment is painful. And you have to live with terrible uncertainty. If ever a person needed courage, this is it.

My friend is a wonderful, optimistic woman. But she hates complaining. Her first instinct was to keep her scared feelings to herself. Unfortunately, that meant that she'd be alone with them and they would fester and destroy her emotional energy.

My friend's instinctive wisdom came to the rescue. She knew that this was one time in her life when she couldn't go it alone. So she cried and complained to her husband, family, and friends. She revealed her sad, scared feelings so she could get all the reassurance it was possible to get from the people who cared about her. That reassurance gave her courage. Courage gave her energy. And she made it all happen by doing what comes naturally to all of us.

When you need courage, you have to reach out to others in any way you can. Why do you think they invented solitary confinement? Because it breaks people's spirits. Isolation is a recipe for emotional exhaustion.

Diagnostic Question #13

Do you have people you regularly talk to honestly about all the things in your life that really bother you?

A no answer to this question means that this secret will give you a big boost of emotional energy.

We All Need to Open Up

Maybe you think this doesn't apply to you. You have plenty of friends and acquaintances, to say nothing of family members and maybe a spouse. So you would never be going it alone, would you?

Unfortunately, maybe you would go it alone. All of us do at certain times in our lives. The reason is *shame*. With all of the people in our lives, there are always going to be issues that make us ashamed, and these are precisely the issues that make us feel most emotionally exhausted. And so when we need help the most, we're least likely to ask for it.

There are two reasons why shame drives us into isolation.

Sometimes we don't reach out because we're embarrassed and afraid for having the problem we have. As one woman I talked to put it, "All our friends think we have this really great marriage. My husband's so handsome and charming. But the fact is that he's been getting increasingly angry and abusive toward me. Whom can I tell, though? We've been married for almost ten years. All my good friends now are in couples we're friends with. If I tell them, they'll tell their husbands. Actually, what I'm most afraid of is that they'll hear me complaining about my husband and they'll think about the Ned they see when we're all together and I'll just look crazy. Plus, okay, suppose they do believe me. Maybe they'll stop asking us over. Suddenly we stop having a social life. And then if what I said gets back to Ned, he's even more abusive."

This is a bigger issue than you might think. The next time you're at work, look around the office. See all those people? You'd be amazed at how many of them are protecting themselves or protecting someone else by staying silent about a problem. And in the process they're feeling alone, helpless, stupid, weird, and emotionally fatigued. That's why they're not reaching out.

The second reason we don't reach out is that we don't know whom to reach out to. When your toilet's clogged, you call a plumber. But whom do you call if you're a middle-aged, politically correct college professor who increasingly found his wife physically unattractive because of all the weight she'd put on, and so he'd stopped making love to her and their relationship was descending into an angry standoff? Whom is he going to talk to about his wife getting fat and unattractive to him? He could complain to a buddy, but what could his buddy say? "Jeez, that sucks"? What's the point of that?

And he can't tell his wife because he already knows how sensitive she is and she's already complained about his being critical and controlling. A couples therapist? They'd done that years ago and it helped a little, but this guy felt stupid about going into couples therapy for the sole reason that he hated his wife being fat.

I know. We can all make suggestions to this guy or tell him why he shouldn't be embarrassed to talk to this or that person. But the fact is that he doesn't know whom to turn to.

I have a little rule of thumb. You tell me if you think I'm right in your case. My rule of thumb states that *everyone has at least one problem he feels he can't share with anyone.* What's yours? Come on, you know you have one. Well, that's your secret burden. And the bigger your secret burden, or the more of them you have, the more emotionally exhausting it is.

It's like being lost in the middle of nowhere. You're scared you won't be able to find your way out, and you feel very stupid for having gotten lost. You have too much to deal with by yourself. If you could've dealt with it by yourself, you would've. But you're overwhelmed, and you feel bad about yourself, and almost by definition that's a recipe for emotional exhaustion.

Moving Past Shame and Isolation

The solution may be easier than you thought. That's the difference our understanding of emotional energy makes. When you're ruled by shame or you don't know whom to turn to, you stay stuck with your secret burden because you're not thinking about what it does to your emotional energy. But that would be like going to work in the morning with a forty-pound pack strapped on your back without thinking about what that will do to your physical energy.

Everything changes when you make your emotional energy a priority. Then you realize that every other consideration takes second place to getting more emotional energy. Are you ashamed to tell people about your secret burden? Okay, I understand. But facing your shame is a small price to pay for regaining your emotional energy.

But what are you really so embarrassed about? Having the problem that you have? Everyone has some problem. Don't be so self-centered. When you talk about your problem, the other person's reaction usually is "Oh, now it will be easier for me to talk about *my* problem."

Or are you embarrassed about complaining in the first place? You might be making a mistake in how you think about it. You think it makes you seem weak. But to other people it makes you seem human.

Once you break through, you get huge dividends of support and help. And you know what? At some point you're going to have to reach out in spite of your shame anyway. We all do eventually. So why not do it before you get to the point of emotional exhaustion?

Here's a guy who got into trouble because he tried to go it alone. I'm sure the details of your life are different from his. But here's what *is* similar: You have a problem that makes you feel isolated because you're ashamed of having that problem. And yet there is someone you could go to for help.

Arnie, 34: "How do we get ourselves into these things? It was the toughest period in my life. And everything I did only made it worse. Here's what happened. I'd been on track for making partner in my law firm. You know going in that not everyone is going to make partner. But I'd brought in some business and done well, and I knew people liked me there. At one point one of the partners during an evaluation told me, 'We like what you're doing around here.' It was obviously stupid, looking back, but I read the tea leaves, looked at the competition, and figured I was in.

"Of course I told my wife I was going to make partner. I felt I had to. I know that one of the reasons she married me was that I was going to be a successful lawyer like her father. Then our second kid was coming and we figured we needed a bigger house and so we got in over our heads, but it would've been okay if I'd made partner.

"It was just one of those things. Tough times at the law firm. New policies about the number of new partners. Plus a couple of the associates started bringing in all this amazing new business. I got caught in it. I think it would've been easier if they'd fired me, one of those up-or-out policies. But they gave me a small raise and told me I was welcome to stay on staff.

"I was devastated. They said maybe a partnership would materialize in the future for me, but that was just hot air. So what do I do? Tell my wife that I was never going to be the kind of guy her father was? No way.

"I did the only thing I could think of. I pretended that none of this had happened. When she asked about what was happening on the partnership front, I just said things were going slowly, but they looked okay. I didn't tell any of my friends either, because they knew my wife, or their wives or girlfriends knew my wife. I didn't tell my brothers or sisters for the same reason. I guess I felt that it would come out one day and I'd handle it then, but why rush it? Maybe I'd come up with something better in the meantime.

"And every month when the mortgage payments on the new house came up, it was like watching a ninety-mile-an-hour fastball coming right at your head. There wasn't enough money, and there wasn't going to be.

"I started getting so depressed. I didn't see a way out. I was looking for a job working for a corporation quietly on the side, but it was hard to network without my buddies, and there weren't all that many jobs that would bring my income up to partner level. So I'm thinking I'm trapped. I'm doomed. I'm thinking it's just a matter of time before my wife leaves me.

"So this goes on and I'm getting in worse and worse shape. Then one weekend we had to go to my wife's parents' house for a barbecue. And I'm there the whole time with my dark secret, feeling terrible. At one point after we've eaten, my father-in-law asked me to go along with him on his usual after-dinner walk. And he asks me the usual how-are-things-at-work question. And I say fine. Then he just stunned me. He came right out and said, 'Did you make partner?'

"That was it. There was no way to avoid telling the truth without telling a bald-faced lie. I felt scared and ashamed, like when you're a kid and you have to confess to your father that you've broken his favorite putter. I told him the whole story. I think the relief of letting out the truth—it was like when you blow up a balloon and release it and it flies all around the room. Everything came out. My deception. Money troubles. Failing to find a job. Everything.

"My father-in-law just listened. When I finally ran out of steam he was silent for a while, and then he said, 'It sounds like you're in trouble and need help.' That was it! Exactly! I was in deep shit and needed all kinds of help.

"But that's the point. When you're in trouble, *you need help.* Like, duuuhh. He got that. I didn't. I hadn't. So he started talking to me about what I could do. Options I'd never thought of. Like working for another law firm. I'd just assumed I was damaged goods. How could I go from failing to make partner at one place to being serious partner material somewhere else? Again, this was a situation I was afraid of and ashamed of.

"Anyway, my father-in-law—remember, he's thirty-five years older than me—starts telling me all these stories about guys where it hadn't worked out for them at one law firm and then they went to another one and everything was okay. He said, 'Look, Arnie, you just have to handle these things right. The way you present your case to them isn't that you failed to cut the mustard. It's that you didn't fit into the direction your old firm was taking.' And he told me he'd make some calls. He also told me to talk to my friends. 'Give them an opportunity to do you a favor,' he said. 'Then they'll be feeling you owe them one.'

"He'd been very nice about the whole thing. Then he got kind of stern. 'Now this bullshit about not telling Claudia. She's your wife, for chrissake. You've dug yourself into a hole, but you've got to be a man and find out what kind of person she is. She's my daughter, but you've got to have the right person in the foxhole with you. If she can't come through for you, then you don't want her. But I think I know her. I hope I know her. I know she's ambitious, but I don't think she's all that shallow. Just tell her. She'll be pissed as hell for a while, but then you won't be alone with this.'

"I told Claudia on the drive home once the kids had fallen asleep. It was literally the hardest thing I've ever done. I'd rather have told her I'd been cheating on her, which I would never do. And she was royally pissed. She was mad as hell at me all night. The next day she was still mad, but she was really glad I'd finally told her. She told me point blank that if I ever kept something like that from her again, it would be over between us. I felt so sorry for what I'd done, especially when she started being very supportive and telling me I'd come out of this fine.

"At one point she said something I'd never quite admitted to myself. She said, 'Look, if worse comes to worst, maybe this just means you'll be happier doing something other than being a lawyer. Lots of lawyers go into management or finance.' It felt so good to hear that. It was like I wasn't trapped and alone anymore with this shameful private little disaster of mine.

"It was amazing how different I felt getting help. When you're alone with this stuff, it's like you're pushing a car. You just can't do it. Then other people join you. Together it feels so much easier. People help you. The people you care about want to help you. I think we all need to experience that."

Emotional energy booster #13
Even if you're ashamed, even if you don't know whom to
turn to, go to someone to get help with whatever
problem most troubles you.

Ask friends and family for help. Find professionals. If you don't know whom to go to, ask the people you talk to whom they'd go to. Talk to everyone and anyone. Not everyone will offer help and support. But most people will try, and you'll be surprised at who will provide real help. It can be the support kind of help. Or it can be real solid, practical, proactive help, such as picking up the phone and making a call on your behalf. Don't be ashamed to ask for leads to other people who might be able to help you in concrete ways.

The mistake you've been making is thinking of this problem in terms of protecting yourself from shame. But you have to protect yourself from loss of emotional energy. Experiencing a few moments of embarrassment is a small price to pay for the energy you'll feel when people come on board to help you.

14

Bring Something Beautiful into Your Life

Emotional Energy Booster #14

Take your pick, art or nature—it doesn't matter. For myself, I vote for art. I'd rather look at a beautiful painting than sit on a log in the woods. But I'm probably in the minority in this. Maybe you'd rather listen to real birds than a Mozart string quartet. Maybe the luckiest among us are those who like both. It's all sublime, though, and that's what counts for our emotional energy.

Being surrounded by the ugly and the drab takes a huge toll on people's emotional energy. Take prison inmates, for example. One of the deprivations they experience most keenly is how almost every sight and sound is boring at best, and most are grating.

Diagnostic Question #14

Is there a gray, bland, dull quality somewhere in your life?
A **yes** *answer to this question means that this secret*
will give you a big boost of emotional energy.

What Turns You On?

Emotional energy booster #14
If you want a constant stream of emotional energy,
find a way to hook up as often as possible with whatever you
consider to be beautiful and wonderful and sublime.

The key is discovering what turns you on and making sure you have constant hits of it. The beautiful, wonderful thing you bring into your life could be anything. One woman I knew had a green parrot. Now, there's something spectacular about a beautiful bird swooping through your house and landing on your shoulder. There's something thrilling about making a wild creature almost tame so that it lets you coexist with it. This person didn't know what an important source of emotional energy her bird was for her until it died. Of course, we're all deeply pained by the loss of a pet. But there was an extra dimension to this woman's loss: the loss of a daily hit of wild, natural beauty. For a long time she refused to get a new bird out of loyalty to the friend she'd lost. But when she finally did, her emotional energy rebounded.

Take Joe. You wouldn't look at Joe and think he was arty. And you'd be right. He didn't *hate* music, painting, and poetry—they just didn't turn him on. But he found a way to make beauty a cornerstone of his life.

Joe, 34: "I think we all have this reaction when we discover something that we fall in love with: 'Why didn't I get into this sooner?' That's how I felt about mountain climbing. They actually had a mountain climbing club in my college. I could've started this a long time ago. But I didn't.

"Several years ago, though, I went to visit a buddy of mine who had a summer cottage in the White Mountains of New Hampshire. I was going to spend a few days there, mostly play tennis and golf. He suggested we try climbing this mountain that he'd heard was pretty easy for novices. 'What the hell,' I said.

"It was like reluctantly agreeing to go out on a blind date with a woman you end up falling madly in love with. At first it was really just walking in the woods, when we were at the bottom. But the higher we got, the more excited I got. I don't know how to describe it. It was more than just beautiful views. It was like I was conquering this mountain, but with every step closer to the top the mountain was conquering me. It gave me an overwhelming experience. It was more than just beautiful. It was incredibly dramatic.

"I had to do something like that again immediately. Two days later my buddy and I climbed a higher mountain. Tried to, anyway. It was too hard, and we didn't know what we were doing. Luckily we were smart enough to turn back. You can get killed up there. Anyway, I'm not inter-ested in danger. Danger doesn't turn me on. For me it's all about being in the midst of incredible, overpowering beauty.

"Of course, I was immediately hooked. To make a long story short, I joined a club. Then I really pushed it. Every long weekend I tried to go on a climb. I tried to arrange time off from work to go on climbs all over the world. Don't get me wrong. I don't think I'll ever be more than a really enthusiastic amateur. I'm not trying to break any records. I just want to spend as much time as I can high up on a mountain.

"The surprise is how this carries over. You know, I like my job, but still it's pretty much another day at the office. And some days you get beaten up. But just knowing inside me that I've been up a mountain—something so different, so far beyond being in the office—or knowing that in a couple of weeks I'll be going up a mountain again, it's exciting. It puts everything else in my life in perspective. Office politics don't impress me so much. I'm stronger in myself, happier in myself, because I've got this thing I can plug into, and it keeps my batteries fully charged."

Do mountains leave you cold? That doesn't matter. Joe found the right way for him. What's the right way for *you* to connect to the sublime?

There Are Many Paths to the Sublime

Here are some of the surprising ways people have made the sublime a part of their lives and gotten emotional energy from it.

One woman, when a difficult pregnancy forced her to stay in bed for weeks, took up embroidery. She'd never thought of herself as a "needlework kind of person." It was really more something to give herself a diversion from watching TV all day. But then she got caught up in the sheer beauty of what she could create. And the thrill of making something beautiful from nothing gave her more emotional energy than anything else during this frustrating, worry-filled time when she needed it so desperately.

One man, now a middle-aged banker, had been a talented artist when he was a kid. He'd always drawn and painted, and an art teacher in high school had pushed him to become an artist. But he'd been too practical to want to risk that route. So he set off for a life in business. But he'd thrown the baby out with the bathwater, and he'd done nothing with his talent. One summer, though, his wife finally forced him to take a three-week vacation. The guy was in a panic. What would he do for three weeks at the seashore?

One night he heard something on the History Channel about Churchill being an amateur painter. He remembered his own artistic past, and he felt some desire surge up from the depths. He brought oil paints, canvases, the works, and took them to the shore. He amazed himself and his wife by spending hours every day joyously painting.

Here's what I do. It may not be as creative, but it gives me just as much contact with the sublime. I started this a few years ago and it's now the high point of my day. I wanted to really get to know classical music. So I decided, along with my husband, that we'd go through the entire history of music, starting with medieval music, in chronological order. Every day we'd listen to a piece of music. For every composer we tried to listen to as many compositions as possible. I know: It probably sounds obsessive. And it's going to take us years. But, God, it's been wonderful.

Listening to music in your car while you're driving to work is just not the same thing. The point is to bring the sublime into your life and highlight it. Do something special. Get something special for yourself.

I don't know how to say this more clearly: If you're not doing it now, you need to start doing it today. Figure out what for you is the beautiful and the sublime, and make it your mission to turn that into a major part of your life.

It doesn't necessarily take money, time, or talent. It just requires an understanding that contact with the sublime gives energy. Amy was a poor woman who worked in a factory and lived in a depressing part of town. But she knew she was surrounded by ugliness, and realizing that helped her.

Amy, 41: "I wonder what would've happened if it hadn't rained that day. I think I would've found my way to all this wonderful art somehow. But when the rain started really coming down, I was walking past the library and I ducked inside. I do remember that I'd been thinking about how ugly my neighborhood was.

"So I get into the library and they have these displays of books they're featuring. That day they were art books. They were celebrating something to do with the Renaissance. And I was drawn to those books like those giant magnets they have in cartoons. I was just pulled right over.

"I fell in love with those pictures. I got a library card, took home a couple of books. Every two weeks I would take out a couple of new art books. Just for the pictures. I mean, I'd read too, but really I just cared about the pictures. Every night after I got the kids to bed and cleaned up the kitchen and brushed my teeth, you know, it's that period when you're ready to collapse, but I'd get into bed with all my art books and look at Michelangelo and Raphael and Rembrandt and Titian and Rubens and

Caravaggio—I really liked the Old Masters. It was just me and this incredible art, like I was the richest woman in the world with the greatest private collection and I could look at any painting in the world for as long as I wanted to.

"I guess maybe I have a visual kind of mind, because I'd really remember those paintings. The experience lasted. Sometimes during the day I'd think about some of the paintings I'd seen. Maybe I'd see someone at work and their face would remind me of someone in a painting.

"It was my secret. I never told anyone. Who would I tell? My best girlfriend knew, and she thought it was kind of funny, but if it made me happy, what did she care? But, you know, it made everything different. I'm serious. My life was different because of those great paintings. I just remember once feeling so sad because I thought the life I led was ugly. By looking at those paintings I brought beauty into my life. It gave me hope."

Special Issue:

Night Thoughts

When you're emotionally tired, the demons come out at night.

You put your head on the pillow, but instead of the blessing of sleep the curse of painful thoughts afflicts your poor brain. Worries sprout like weeds. Sadness spreads like red wine spilled on a white tablecloth. If you're lucky enough to fall asleep, maybe you wake up in the middle of the night, and then the night thoughts come out.

Maybe you see very clearly what a financial hole you've dug for yourself and how easy it will be for you to go bankrupt. Or you think about how everything you've wanted most in life you didn't get and probably will never get. You remember with pain some terrible failure or humiliation from ten years ago. You have a deep understanding of how you're a complete self-destructive idiot.

We've all been there. We've all had night thoughts like these and many others.

It's time we acknowledged how wrong this is. The night is not a lens that enables us to peer more deeply into the truth. It's a time of swirling smoke and distorted mirrors that turn seeds of truth into nightmarish shapes.

And night thoughts are terribly unhealthy. They make you afraid to go to bed. They taint the rest you need. And you remember them during the day. They're like waking nightmares with credibility.

Say Goodnight to Night Thoughts

Most people are susceptible to painful night thoughts. Here's how to prevent yourself from falling victim to them.

First, maintain good sleep hygiene. Go to sleep at the same time every night. Don't drink alcohol or caffeine before sleep. Don't go to sleep on a full stomach. Make sure your bedroom is comfortable, dark, and well ventilated. Eating a small amount of complex carbohydrates (like a slice of bread or a couple of cookies or crackers) can help you fall asleep. Follow a restful routine before you go to bed, like taking a bath or reading a book.

Second, develop a list of things to think about that will help you fall asleep. Here are some proven suggestions—and you can also come up with some of your own.

- Play tennis or golf games in your head.
- Remember all the people you've ever known.
- Remember your favorite songs and sing them to yourself.
- List all the books you've loved.
- List all the states with their capitals.
- Imagine all the places you'd like to see.
- Remember all the places you've lived or visited.
- Try to remember in detail the last movie you saw.
- List all the famous people you can think of.
- See yourself going on your favorite walks.
- *Visualize yourself having emotional energy when you do whatever it is you're going to do tomorrow.*

A little trick many people have is to use the alphabet to make lists. Whatever it is you're trying to list—friends, countries, famous people, whatever—try to think of one for each letter of the alphabet in order. Australia, Brazil, Colombia . . . you get the picture. There's something very boring and yet engrossing about doing this. It puts you to sleep, but it prevents you from thinking about anything else.

Whatever you think about, the point is to think of some pocket of life that's interesting to you, familiar, and pleasurable. Then think about it in such a way that you can keep your mind occupied for a chunk of time.

It's a fact: Some things are painful to think about, and some things are pleasurable or relaxing to think about. Take responsibility for having good thoughts to substitute for bad thoughts at night. You'd be amazed at how effective this is, but you have to make yourself do it.

The third thing to do, if night thoughts overwhelm you, is to get out of bed and go read a book or magazine. Eat a small amount of carbohydrates. Don't read for much more than half an hour. The minute you feel yourself getting a little sleepy, go back to bed. You'll almost certainly find it's easier to go to sleep without bad thoughts.

What you're doing is teaching yourself that you won't put up with painful night thoughts. You have better things to think about. Somehow this no-tolerance policy gives the part of you that produces night thoughts the message that it should give up and stop bothering you. Then you're free.

15

Fire Your Critics, Gloom Merchants, and Naysayers

Emotional Energy Booster #15

What's the most important form of wealth? Money is nice, of course. Real estate is good. But for most of us our greatest wealth comes from the people in our lives. Love, friendship, community, kindness, fun, support, connections, future projects—all these grow out of our friends and family. And because people are so important, we tend to fill our lives with them, like an art collector filling his house with all the paintings he can lay his hands on.

But here's another question. What's the greatest irritant in your life? Work? Pollution? Sore feet? Maybe, but for many of us the most pervasive and deepest irritant is some of the people in our lives.

People Pollution Is the Worst Pollution

There's nothing worse than obnoxious, draining, frustrating, infuriating people who seem to suck the life out of you. People who put you down. People who bum you out. People who take more than they give.

People who waste your time. People who hurt you. People with whom you have nothing in common. And everyone has people like this in their lives.

Here's what some men and women have said to me:

- "I have ideas for things I want to do—little things, like taking a trip or buying something for the kitchen—but whatever it is that I want to do, my boyfriend tells me that it's a bad idea."

- "I have this friend at work who always begins talking to me by saying, 'You know what's wrong with you? . . .' She's a little older than me, and I know, at least I think, that she's trying to be help-ful, but she always makes me feel that I don't have the right stuff."

- "I have this successful brother who's always making me do what he wants me to do. Like if he thinks we should go in together on a summer rental, he bullies me until I agree with him, and then he makes me feel like a big idiot for not having seen it his way all along. He's the most controlling person I know."

- "There's this woman who's one of my oldest friends. We were roommates for three years in college, and we were very close. But in the past ten years things have changed a lot. I'm doing fine in my life and I'm having a lot of fun. She's having one self-inflicted disaster after another. And she's always suffering and complaining and asking me to let her stay with me or lend her money or just listen by the hour to her problems. I feel very guilty, but this relationship is a total drain."

- "My father is such a drag on my life. Whatever I want to do, he starts worrying about it and telling me how things could go wrong. Let's say I want to buy an SUV. He starts talking about the low gas mileage and how SUVs tip over. So I say I'll buy a sedan. 'Yeah,' he says, 'but what about the resale value?' There's always something wrong with everything I want to do. It's exhausting."

Show me someone suffering from emotional exhaustion and I'll find someone in that person's life who saps their energy. We usually act as if people like this were a minor annoyance. But in fact they're a disaster.

Diagnostic Question #15

Are there people in your life who more often than not leave you feeling worse when you interact with them?

A **yes** *answer to this question means that this secret will give you a big boost of emotional energy.*

If we want to maintain our emotional energy, we have to identify the people who drain us. And we have to loosen our ties to them, if only a little. The good news is that there are often huge payoffs in emotional energy from stepping back ever so slightly from a critic or gloom merchant.

Ending People Pollution

First you have to identify the people who emotionally exhaust you.

The easy part is knowing who the worriers, naysayers, fear-mongers, guilt-makers, and finger-pointers are: When you find you're about to talk to one of them, your immediate reaction is "Yecccccchhhhh!" The hard part is admitting that these people are more trouble than they're worth. We make excuses. We explain why they do what they do. We put on blinders. We go into denial. We say, "Yeah, she's very negative and no fun at all, but she means well and we've been friends for a long time."

But what the heck is that saying? It's saying what we all say in a situation like this. "This friend/lover/relative is a big drain on me, but I don't want to see myself as anything other than loyal and well intentioned."

Okay, you're a good person. But I can't believe you think your goodness extends to letting yourself be eaten alive. Here's the truth. You have a limited amount of energy. The people who drain it prevent you from giving to the people you care about. It's not goodness to let people you care about less take from people you care about more. They're stealing your life.

Gloria, 34: "People look at me and think, 'Oh, she's this cute little hair-dresser.' What they don't see is that I have all kinds of talent and dreams and ambitions. I studied hairdressing and I practiced and I entered competitions. One day I knew I would go to Los Angeles and be a hairdresser for movie stars and like that. But, you know, my friends started trying to bust me. They were like, 'Gloria, all this stuff you talk about, what makes you think that you can make it out there when there are a million girls like you?' And the truth was, I got scared. I knew what to do. I knew how to do it. I was ready. But I couldn't pull myself together to make it happen. I was losing my push. I was getting worn out before I started. It's like I'd gone missing on myself.

"And then I realized how much it was getting to me, all that stuff my friends were saying. I'd been thinking, 'They're my friends; they're trying to help me.' And I know they'd do anything for me. But come on, they're trying to help themselves. They don't see themselves making a big move like I want to make. So they have to justify to themselves what they're doing. This stuff they're staying to me to make me feel bad about thinking of going makes them feel good about thinking of staying.

"But I have this aunt—she's my mother's older sister. I've always looked up to her. She asked me about my plans, and I told her about how I was getting afraid. She told me how you'll never do anything really good if you don't do the things you want to do because of fear. You can't let your fear hold you back. I got so much energy from that. So I made my plans, and now I'm all set to go."

I had an image of Gloria's friends siphoning off fuel from her fuel tank so that she started running on empty, and then her aunt suddenly giving her a big injection of high-octane fuel. Fuel. That's what emotional energy is. You can't let people take it away from you.

Say Bye-bye to the Bad Guys

You've taken the hard step: identifying the people who take so much emotional energy from you that they're more trouble than they're worth.

The next step is easy. Imagine that you and the other person are connected by a rope. Now let go of the rope a little bit. Not completely. Just a small step back. The next time they talk about getting together, say no. If you do get together, leave early. Schedule less time together. And step back emotionally too. Don't talk about your most intimate realities. If the other person talks about intimate details, don't be so eager to participate.

A big brother or sister who's a bully? Have less to do with that person. A troublemaking coworker? Ignore him or her more than you've been doing. A worry-monger? Don't tell such a person things to worry about.

Do what Gloria did. Edge away from people who are stealing your energy by edging closer to people who give you energy.

It's not the distance you create that gives you back your energy. It's doing something to create that distance that gives you energy. One less phone call a week isn't that big a deal. But the fact that you've done something to take back a small piece of your life, that's where you get a surge.

And here's why. When you let your energy be cannibalized, you know you're facing a future that's draining, and that's what exhausts you. But when you do something to edge away, you build a whole new relationship of trust with yourself. You're saying, "Self, now I can trust you to take care of me, because you've shown me that you can let go of emotional cannibals." Taking a small step away can pay big dividends in self-trust, which pays even bigger dividends in your emotional energy.

Emotional energy booster #15
Don't give your precious emotional energy to people who drain your emotional energy. Step back from them any way you can.

16

Life Is Too Important to Take Too Seriously

Emotional Energy Booster #16

Suppose you could design the universe. Would you design it as a grim place or a fun place? Fun, of course. Let's face it, that's how we want the universe to be.

And yet that's not how we actually live. For most of us day-to-day reality is filled with decisions and responsibilities that are overwhelming. Deadlines. Goals we have to meet. People we have to satisfy. They suck the energy right out of us.

Even happy events get tainted with this. How many times have we seen that planning a wedding or the arrival of a baby turns into a grim experience? Something that should be fun is tainted by the fear of making a mistake.

I know one woman who's a real estate broker and a mother. She likes showing houses to people. She likes playing with her children. But when it comes to talking to people about actually buying a house, she always feels her entire career is on the line. And although she could enjoy herself with her kids, she's so upset about their performance in school that their future always seems in jeopardy to her.

It's as if her life were a high-stakes poker game where she just bet her mortgage money and she knows she's not holding winning cards. *That's* a recipe for emotional exhaustion, and that's how many people approach their lives. It's not a game, it's a knife to their throat.

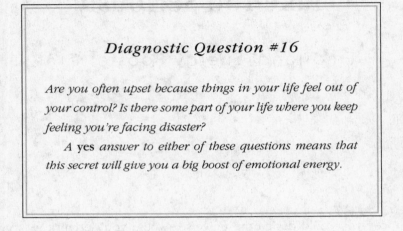

Diagnostic Question #16

Are you often upset because things in your life feel out of your control? Is there some part of your life where you keep feeling you're facing disaster?

A **yes** *answer to either of these questions means that this secret will give you a big boost of emotional energy.*

High-energy people live the same life you and I do. The same pressures. The same concerns. It's not their special life that gives them energy. It's that they bring energy to their lives. How? They have a special approach to life that saves their emotional energy when they're under the gun. Let me tell you what this approach is and how you can adopt it yourself.

"It Just Doesn't Matter"

Do you remember the Bill Murray summer-camp movie *Meatballs*? It's just a fun flick, but there's one small scene in it that can change your life if you know what to do with it. It's the night before the big athletic contest with the other camp. Defeat and doom seem inevitable. Everyone's nervous and bummed out. Their emotional energy is draining in front of our eyes.

Murray makes a speech. His goal is to take the pressure off. The centerpiece of his speech is the passionate refrain "It just doesn't matter! *It just doesn't matter!*" Over and over, louder and louder, he says this, and he gets the kids to join him until everyone's shouting it at the top of their lungs.

A crazy thing for him to do? Murray's speech is actually a very smart move. It's fun to win. It's fun to play. But when you're afraid you're going to lose, energy gets lost at an alarming rate. The more we think that what we do matters immensely, the more we choke and panic and suffer. All joy is lost. People who live as if they're on the verge of disaster have no possibility of fun, and so they're cut off from emotional energy.

The secret is to stop taking things so seriously. I'll show you how to do this in a moment. But I know that right now this may seem impossible to you. "My reality is grim—I've got to take it extremely seriously." Well, your reality may be grim, but you *don't* have to take it so seriously.

Laughing Through Scary Times

I've lived through plenty of scary times myself. I spent the first four years of my life in refugee camps. I came to America as a little immigrant girl speaking not a word of English. There was the time as a graduate student when my kids were one and three, we had two hundred dollars in the bank with no income and no prospect of any money soon, and our families weren't able to help us out. I've lived through thinking my husband was about to die. I've lived through a breast cancer scare. I've lived through a mysterious condition that made me feel my body was falling apart. I've flown on planes the day after a major terrorist attack.

Beyond that, for thirty years I've shared in the difficult and scary times my patients have lived through. I know what it's like to experience the worst that life has to offer.

But I know one other thing. Take two people. Both of them are dealing with the very same difficult situation—whatever situation you want to imagine. What I know is that *they have a choice* about how seriously they will take this situation, and I know that *whoever takes the situation less seriously will have more emotional energy.*

Let's take one of the most difficult situations human beings have ever found themselves in: Auschwitz. The people who did the best job of surviving psychologically were the ones who found ways to take what they were going through less seriously. They joked. They made friends and found ways to enjoy being with their friends. They found ways to entertain themselves. They accepted the fact that they couldn't control whether they lived or died.

Of course, conditions were still grim. You can't go through Auschwitz and psych yourself into thinking that you're living through a garden party. But people could choose to take what they were going through *less* seriously, and when they did they had much more emotional energy.

One of the great books about human endurance, Slavomir Rawicz's *The Long Walk,* is the story of six prisoners who escaped from a Soviet slave labor camp in Siberia and walked four thousand miles over tundra, desert, and mountains until they found safety. You can imagine how grim that was. But Rawicz says that the one quality they appreciated, valued, and needed the most was the ability to make jokes about what they were enduring. He is specifically saying that emotional survival was the key to physical survival, and that the key to emotional survival was emotional energy, and that the key to emotional energy was the ability to not take things so seriously.

Emotional energy booster #16
You can always take what you're going through
a little less seriously. And every time you do
you'll get a big payback in energy.

You take things seriously because you're afraid. Fear is a natural emotion, but it's also an unhealthy one. It's good for animals, because it activates them. Once they're activated, they're not thinking. But they don't need to think. They go by instinct. And since animals don't sit around imagining how tomorrow's going to turn out, their fear never curdles into depression.

It's different for people. Fear makes us stupid and miserable. In the face of any threat you can imagine, the person who's less afraid is smarter and happier. No one would ever choose fear as a good way to deal with a situation. You might wish you'd paid more attention to certain risks, but that's just about being smarter. You'd never wish you'd actually been more afraid.

And yet every time you take things seriously, you're embracing fear, as if that nightmare were your friend. But when you stop taking things so seriously, you heal your relationship with the universe. You do this by seeing the universe as a better place. By taking things less seriously, you actually make the universe a better place. Think of the power you hold in your hands!

When you take things just a little less seriously, you enormously empower yourself. Take a trivial example. You show up for a doctor's appointment and she keeps you waiting. This makes some people succumb to rage and frustration. But by doing so they give away all their power. They let an unimportant circumstance determine how they'll feel. But if you decide to not take waiting so seriously, you show yourself that you're the one who controls how you feel. And that will give you a big hit of emotional energy.

How to Do It

The simplest way to lift yourself out of the trap of taking things too seriously is to straightforwardly use the Bill Murray approach. Think about something in your life that's sucking the emotional energy right out of you. I know it's a big deal. I understand. But tell yourself it just doesn't matter. Let go of your sense of the overwhelming seriousness of it all. Whether things turn out one way or another, you will still be all right.

Some people, when they hear this, are able to flip a switch. They see that they can't keep going the way they've been. If they keep on making a big deal about things, they're going to go down the tubes emotionally.

For many of us it's not so easy. We try to tell ourselves it just doesn't matter, but we find it matters a lot. The reason we're stuck is that it's hard to let go of something when you don't have anything to replace it. So here's what some people do who are successful at not taking things so seriously: They find something else to embrace that fills them with hope, not doom. Fun, not grimness. Pleasure, not pain. Meaning, not emptiness.

And here are the ways they did that.

Embrace the Present

One way to stop taking things so seriously is to embrace today, not tomorrow. You're losing emotional energy because you're focusing on how things will turn out in the future. You'll gain emotional energy when you focus on the present moment. What are you doing right now? How does it feel? How can you make it feel better right now? How would you make this moment that you're in right now better?

Maybe you'd be kinder. Maybe you'd be more focused. But one thing is for sure. If you didn't worry about how this moment was going to turn out, you'd be more relaxed, you wouldn't take it so seriously, you'd enjoy yourself more, and you'd end up making the best of this moment.

You *have* to live in the present. It's the only place where you can make anything good happen. And it's the only place where you can actually enjoy yourself.

Frank, 43: "It was about a year ago that I found out I had ulcers. The message I got came through loud and clear: I was slowly killing myself. Up until then I'd always blamed it on my life, which I admit is pretty demanding. I sell computer systems, which is very competitive, plus I'm always on the road. My boss is demanding. My customers are demanding. Then I have a wife who likes things just so. And my kids are great, but one isn't doing so well in school and the other does well but also acts out a lot. So everywhere I look there are problems.

"But the thing is, it was me. Everything I faced I treated like hand-to-hand combat. Kill or be killed. If my boss read the riot act to me, I was facing doom. If a customer was unhappy, I was facing doom. If my kids got in trouble, they were going right down the tubes.

"And this was all just eating me up inside, literally. I'd get up every morning utterly exhausted. I'd have to drink cup after cup of coffee to keep myself going. I lived on energy bars, and still I had no energy.

"I went out for a drink with a friend after work one Friday and started complaining about everything, and I know I must've made everything seem so damned serious. I'm going on and on, and suddenly my friend breaks in and says, 'Look, you're a good salesman, you're a good husband, you're a good father. So what are you worried about? *Enjoy the ride.*'

"That was it. I could enjoy my life if I focused on living my life. I like selling—if you're a salesman, you understand what I'm talking about. So if I like it and I'm good at it, why not enjoy it? I'll do my best, and whatever happens happens.

"The turning point came when I was talking to a major customer. This guy was big for me. His reorders and upgrades were a large part of my business. He started getting on me about the price of this and the delivery date of that and the specifications for something else. I started getting uptight. But then I remembered I'd better enjoy the ride. So I found myself saying to him, 'Look, we're a good company, you're a good company, things have always worked out. You know I'll do my best for you, and whatever happens happens, but it'll turn out okay.' I just decided inside not to take things so seriously. He looked at me and then he said, 'Yeah, that's right.'

"I still work hard. I still care. But I focus on what's in front of me, in the moment. That's where the fun is, and that's where I get a lot of energy."

What Frank's saying is that life should be the way Little League should be. You play hard, but you enjoy yourself and don't worry about winning. It's all about the game, not the score. The game is in the present, and the score is all about a future you can't touch.

Focus on Yourself

Another way high-energy people found to stop taking things so seriously was to focus on themselves, not on other people. You have needs, feelings, thoughts, dreams. If you focus on what's happening for you and on what you need, the things other people are doing will become less important.

This is not the same as being selfish. But when the ten most important people in your life are all making demands on you, you'll feel overwhelmed unless you ask yourself what you want.

Mandy, 36: "I'm a freelance journalist who mostly writes about people who've gone through some kind of catastrophe, sometimes recently, sometimes a long time ago. I used to worry a lot about the people I wrote about. They often had so many problems, and I'd always be afraid of what would happen to them in the future. I felt I was carrying all these fragile lives around in my hands, and my hands were trembling.

"When I'd interview them, I'd look at the person sitting across from me like he or she was a bomb that could go off at any moment. Of course, I got to the point pretty fast where I stopped wanting to go to work. It was all far too exhausting.

"Then I realized that I was letting myself be traumatized by their traumas, and I was losing myself the way trauma victims sometimes do. I don't know how I came to this insight, but I decided to focus on myself.

"I decided to take care of myself. So I turned the energy I'd used up monitoring them to monitoring myself. Was I happy sitting here with this other person? Focused? Safe? Let's say I was bored. If so, maybe we were getting stuck going over the same information. If I shook things up a bit, at least I wouldn't be bored.

"I got so many benefits from this. For example, I'd been a painter in my spare time, and I felt there'd been a limp, halfhearted, low-energy quality in my pictures for a long time. But that's because I wasn't there. I was worried about how the painting on the canvas would turn out, and I wasn't thinking about what was going on inside me that I wanted to paint.

When you paint a painting, you're telling a story even if it's abstract. But what was my story? When I focused on myself, I got in touch with the pieces of the stories I wanted to tell, and that reexcited me when it came to doing my painting."

This solution works because part of the process of taking things too seriously is getting caught up in thinking about what other people want. That puts you in a state of overload. You're taking care of too many people. Focusing on yourself is a way to make things easier on yourself.

Have Perspective

Another way people found to stop taking things so seriously is they stopped focusing on the minutiae and paid more attention to the big picture.

Danny, 49: "I recently started my fourth term in Congress. As a Democrat, I've found it frustrating to be in the minority. A few years ago I realized that I saw my entire political life as a series of battles, and I was desperate to win each one, as if the balance of the future were in doubt. So there'd be these little bills and amendments—yes, they were all important to someone and worth being taken seriously, but they didn't have to be taken all that seriously. I didn't see that at the time, though.

"We went to a party conference at one point and a speaker mentioned that we politicians were there to make the world a better place. Now, that may seem to you like a lame thing to say. Doesn't every commencement speaker say something like that? But it got through to me big time. I saw that that was the first line of my job description. I was in Congress to make the world a better place. That was my fight. That was my issue.

"I worked as hard as I did before. Maybe harder. I'm more hopeful now. Happier. And it's because I don't take every bill, every vote, so damned seriously. We're all here to make the world a better place. And we will. I'm going to win some and I'm going to lose some, but we are going to move the ball down the field. I know I'm going to leave the world better than I found it. So why do I have to get all upset in the meantime? The rest is details."

Come on. Is it going to change your child's future whether or not you give him a little extra help with his homework tonight? Is this something that makes all the difference between successful adults and failures? Is it going to spoil your high school reunion that you've only lost ten pounds and not the twenty pounds you were hoping to lose? I could go on and on with these examples. But you and I know that if you said about everything you take seriously, "Does this really matter in the long run?" you'd say no nine times out of ten. And then you'd have perspective. Then you'd have fun and you'd relax. And then you'd have a lot more emotional energy.

It's Up to You

So that's how you stop taking things so seriously. Focus on the moment, not the future. Focus on yourself, not on what's going on around you. Focus on what's most important in the big picture, not on petty little issues. You can do this everywhere in your life.

When you take things too seriously, your energy leaks out into a future where you're not even present. When you stop taking things so seriously, you save all your emotional energy for right now, which is when you need it.

17

Clear the Decks

Emotional Energy Booster #17

Diagnostic Question #17

Are there important parts of your life that feel up in the air to you? Do you feel overwhelmed with all the things you think you have to do? Do you feel you're busy with a lot of stuff that doesn't mean very much to you?

*A **yes** answer to any of these questions means that this secret will give you a big boost of emotional energy.*

Two runners. The first is carrying around a lot of junk with him. The second is unencumbered. The first is confused about whether he should be running at all. The second knows that he's doing exactly what he wants to do. Who wins the race?

I don't know. Maybe the first guy is a great runner. But I do know this: The second guy will have a lot more energy and will feel a lot better throughout the race.

So—do you have emotional energy? If not, maybe the problem is clutter, the kind of clutter that makes us emotionally exhausted.

There are lots of ways our lives get cluttered and lots of ways to get rid of the clutter and give ourselves a big energy boost. Let's start with just one of these ways and then move on to others.

Just Decide, Damn It

Let's say that for a long time now you've been talking about getting your hair cut really short. It will look good, you think. But will it be too extreme? It will be fashionable. But will it suit you? You have long conversations with your friends about whether to get your hair cut short or not.

You're thinking about the best thing to do, and I say forget it. If you want more emotional energy, *just do it*. Get on the phone right now, make the first available appointment, and damn it, go get your hair cut short. *Or just let go of it*. If you'd really wanted to do it, you'd have done it. You don't want it. So stop talking about it.

I don't give a damn how short your hair will be. *You* probably don't care that much when you really think about it. You just want to look good.

But that decision hanging over your head—it's been sucking the life out of you. So what do you do? You let go of everything except the need to put this decision behind you once and for all.

High-energy people make a decision and move on. The emotionally exhausted stay stuck, unable to decide. And the more unmade decisions they're dragging around, the more burdened they are and the more emotionally exhausted they are.

Every time you can't make a decision, you're burdening yourself with all the alternatives you can't let go of. You're carrying around the short-haired you and the long-haired you. The you that's moved to California and the you that hasn't. The you that's got a dog and the you that doesn't.

At every turn your burden doubles. The more unmade decisions in your life, and the more important these decisions are, the greater the burden.

David, 38: "I sometimes feel there's something very wrong with me for being in this situation, very weird. It's hard for me to imagine that other people's lives are as much up in the air as mine. I hope they're not. But sometimes I'm afraid there are a lot of people like me.

"Here's my dilemma. I'm a programmer; I make an okay living. But even if I get promoted, I'm not going to make lots of money or move to a high corporate level. This was always okay with me, because I liked my work, but I've been getting antsy. There are bigger horizons out there careerwise. I could move into sales. I could move into management.

"One thing that's gotten clear to me is that in my field there are more opportunities out on the West Coast. So if I want to move up, it would help to move west. But that's a big deal. My family's here, and so is my wife's. They'd be upset if we moved. In a way that's a plus, though, because our families have been so involved with us, it's driving us crazy.

"But Sally, my wife, and I get to talking about moving to California, or at least looking for work out there, and just when we're all excited about going, we get scared about the risk and the expense and we start thinking about what we're going to miss from our lives here in Boston. So then we backtrack. It's as if our whole future keeps staying up in the air because we don't know what we want to be when we grow up or where we want to live.

"Now, that's all bad enough. But Sally wants to get pregnant. Again. We have two sons, but she really wants a daughter. She's two years older than me, so she's really feeling it's got to be now or never. Mostly she wants it to be now, but sometimes she gets scared and says to forget it. I've been very clear—I don't want any more children. I'm just getting happy with the thought that my kids have reached the age where they can take care of themselves. I'm needing to take care of myself now. I don't need a baby.

"But mostly Sally pushes and pushes on the baby thing. So between us we're completely undecided. I guess, though, I have a secret that plays in here. It's no accident that she's grabbing hold of this baby thing. Our marriage hasn't been happy for a while. We've grown apart. Sally's a teacher and doesn't care about what I do for a living. We don't talk about anything except the kids and these stupid decisions that are weighing on us.

"But once when we were talking she said, kind of jokingly, that if I just got her pregnant and took off for Silicon Valley and left her in Boston, she'd be very happy. 'You're the one who wants to move,' she said.

"The worst part of it is how all these decisions are tangled up together. If we have a baby, it's harder to move. If I change careers, it's better to move. If we don't have a baby, will we stay together? If we don't stay together, then why shouldn't I move? Except she'd probably stay in Boston and then I'd want to be here, otherwise I'd never see my sons.

"Can you follow all of this? It's hard for me to follow it most of the time. All I know is that I'm a wreck. I can't sleep. I'm not doing my job. And I'm turning into this gloomy, burned-out guy. The really scary part is the more exhausted I am by all this, the harder it is to deal with. And the more I don't deal with it, the harder it all gets and the more down I feel."

We're all burdened by unmade decisions. How do we break through the impasse and move on?

There are two main reasons we get stuck. First, we think we need to make a very high-quality decision. Not just a good decision, but a smart, brilliant, excellent decision. Second, we experience our decisions as being all tangled up with one another. You can see that with David. But even if all you're thinking about is getting a haircut, maybe that's tangled up with whether you want to buy a lot of new clothes, with whether you're thinking about dumping your boyfriend, with whether or not this woman at work who's been really bugging you is also going to get a short haircut, and who knows what else.

The burdens of wanting to make a great decision and of one decision being tangled up with a bunch of others completely paralyze us. We forget one simple thing. *Nothing is more important than emotional energy. Nothing destroys emotional energy like a backlog of unmade decisions.*

Once you realize that the most important thing is getting more emotional energy, all you'll want to do is make your damned decision, get the energy boost, and move on.

Here's what happened to David. No one could have been more surprised than he at how quickly his burden was lifted. Let's revisit him a few months later.

David: "It's funny how things happen. Sally was crying about wanting a daughter. 'It's all I've ever wanted,' she said. 'I know there's only a fifty-fifty chance, but I just want a chance.' I suddenly felt very cruel and mean for not giving that to her. It felt stupid for me to leave this issue up in the air between us. One more kid. What's the big deal? But it really matters to Sally.

"So I said yes, okay, absolutely. She couldn't believe it that I suddenly caved in, because I'm very stubborn, but of course she was ecstatic. I'd thought I'd be kind of depressed, but what I felt most was relief. The key thing was that this was *settled*. That's what I kept telling myself. We've settled this. It was like a weight was taken off my shoulders.

"Then everything fell into place. Once I decided we'd try to have another child, I decided to stop thinking about divorcing Sally. Then moving to the West Coast seemed a more difficult thing to do, so I decided the hell with it. If I get an offer out there, we'll see, but I'm not going to look for it. And then I decided that I liked being a computer programmer. Yes, there was a ceiling, but I could keep upgrading my skills, and at least I'd know I was doing something I was good at and that I enjoyed.

"It's amazing how fast my life went from being completely up in the air to being completely settled. I'd thought I'd feel terrible. Afraid I was trapped. Afraid I'd made a horrible mistake. But I just felt great. Sally told me in the weeks afterward that I'd become a good guy again, someone she wanted to be around. I started feeling I wanted to be around myself too."

Make *any* decision. It doesn't have to be the biggest decision that's weighing on you these days. Decide what you're going to eat tonight.

Then decide whether you're going to buy that CD or not. Then decide about your haircut. Then make a decision about your future.

In decision land, all this stuff can seem very important. In emotional energy land, ending your ambivalence and making a good-enough decision is what's important. A decision a day keeps the doctor away.

But unmade decisions are just one form of clutter. The real issue is the stuff in your life that snags your attention, wastes your time, and drains your emotional energy.

Cluttered Lives Kill Emotional Energy

One of the most striking things you notice about people who have a lot of emotional energy is how streamlined their minds and lives are. Sure, their desks might be buried under messy piles of papers, but in truth they don't waste time with things that aren't important to them. That's why it's so important to make decisions. You deal with something and move on.

Unfinished business saps energy. It's emotional clutter. And there are all kinds of unfinished business. Items on your to-do list that you neither need nor want to do are part of it. But people too can be a form of clutter—if they are people you don't need in your life who take energy away from you without giving you energy back.

> ### Emotional energy booster #17
> *Get rid of the unfinished business in your life. Just deal with it one way or another. Finish it or forget about it. Make a decision. If you do this, you'll get more emotional energy.*

Ricki was someone I approached because she seemed to be bubbling with high emotional energy. I wanted to know her secret. What she told me was how she'd recently gotten out of a low-energy state.

Ricki, 34: "You know how sometimes you run into an old friend and she asks if you're in a relationship? I guess you know you're in trouble if you don't have a clue how to answer, not even to yourself.

"That was me with Nick. Not in a committed relationship. Available but not looking. Wanting to be in love. Seeing him off and on for years. Sometimes we'd go out, sometimes we'd have sex, sometimes we'd talk about other relationships, sometimes we'd toy with the idea of our being a couple.

"What is all that? A lot of junk. So who was Nick to me? You tell me. I didn't know what we had or where we were going. All we had was a comfort factor. One day Nick tells me about a woman at work that he was having 'feelings' for. It was the kind of conversation we'd had dozens of times. Two hours earlier we'd made love. Now we're buddies or something. I felt sick of the messiness of the whole thing. The up-in-the-airness of it all.

"I can't believe what I said. I just said, 'Nick, listen. Ask me to marry you right now or we're over.' Boom. Like that. And he hesitated way past that point, you know, where you know he's not going to ask you to marry him. So I just said, 'Okay, then we're over.' That was it. Bye-bye.

"I thought I'd be sad and scared, but I felt fantastic. I'd thought Nick was giving me something in my life. But what he really was doing was clogging up my life. I'll tell you something. If it's not right for you, it's wrong for you. Nick was wrong for me because he wasn't right for me. For the first time in years I felt hopeful about meeting someone who was right for me."

We're All Drowning in Unfinished Business

There are people you can hire to come into your physical space—your closets, your drawers, your desktop—and clean it out, getting rid of everything that's not necessary, organizing what's left.

We need something like this for our inner space even more. All the things you have to do and want to do but haven't gotten around to. All the projects you've started and haven't finished. All the people and activities that don't really add anything to your life.

If you want a big, fast hit of energy, you have to clean out this clutter from your life. I'll admit it's not easy to get rid of the people and activities that sap our energy. Here's an analogy. Take your closet. It's filled with clothes that are too small . . . but maybe you'll be able to fit into them one day. It's filled with clothes you don't like anymore . . . but maybe the perfect occasion for wearing them will turn up. It's filled with clothes that need mending . . . but maybe one day you'll have the time to sit down and sew on buttons.

Maybe you will . . . but probably you won't. Meanwhile you're weighed down and clogged up with clutter.

The Appointment-Book Cure

Let me tell you about an amazing way out of the clutter trap.

Everyone has some kind of to-do list and some kind of appointment book that govern their lives. For most there are many to-do lists. There's a do-today list that you may just carry around in your head. There's a must-do list that maybe you've written down on your desk—these are often top-priority items. There's an important-things-to-do list that's stashed away somewhere but gives you heartache whenever you think of it.

Then there's your appointment book. This could be anything from a Palm Pilot or a date book to a calendar or even a piece of paper you have on the fridge reminding you to do something at a particular time that day.

Now here's how to get rid of the unfinished business in your life. *Never, ever have a to-do list of any sort. If something comes up for you to do, put it in your appointment book in a specific time slot. Eventually all the things you have to do in your life will only be in your appointment book.* Everyone who does this feels an immediate surge of emotional energy.

Let's say that on your to-do list you have "Call Cousin Ruthie to ask her if she's bringing a date to the wedding." Go to your appointment book and find a time to call Ruthie. Maybe you'll write it down for Saturday morning at ten. Now you have an appointment to do it. If Ruthie isn't home and you can't leave a message, write down another time in your book to call her. The point is to be controlled by your appointment book. *That's* how you get yourself to get rid of the unfinished business in your life.

Let's say that on your to-do list you have "Pull together a new résumé."

This is obviously a big task. You may have no idea how long it will take or even what's involved in completing the task. But that's okay. Go to your appointment book and block out four hours in which all you'll do is work on your résumé. You'll get as much done as you can in four hours. It may be a lot. You may just end up with a lot of questions. That's okay too. Then go to your appointment book and block out another chunk of time in which you'll take the next step.

The point is that it all has to be controlled by *when* you do it, not by *what* you do. By focusing on *when,* you've completely gotten rid of the emotionally draining overhang of things to do. Either there's a time for it, or there's no time for it and it's gone.

Let's say you have a letter from your alumni association on your desk. It will soon be your tenth reunion. They want you to write them what you've been doing since college and send them some money. Your mind boggles. How can you possibly summarize what you've been doing since college? How can you possibly figure out how much money to send them? Aaarrrrrgggggghhhhh! It's too hard to deal with right away. It's too important to get rid of. So it's just been sitting there on your desk, which is really a visible to-do list, cluttered with things that remind you by virtue of their physical presence that you have to do them.

That stupid letter, like all the things you have to do, is doing its share to drain your emotional energy. Transfer dealing with it from your to-do list to your appointment book. Maybe that means doing it right now. Maybe that means putting it down for Sunday evening when you have an appointment to clear away a lot of paperwork. Maybe that means just throwing the damn letter away.

Sometimes the Best Thing to Do with Clutter Is Throw It Away

Think about that last idea for a moment. All those items on your to-do list—if you don't want to make a specific time to do them, that's your way of saying you don't want to do them at all. And that's fantastic. The best way to deal with any of those things you might at one time have put on your to-do list is to throw them away and never do them. Nothing is easier and faster than *not* doing something.

If you're not going to do something, set it free. Set yourself free from it. Annihilate it from your life and your consciousness. Give yourself the explosion of energy that comes from saying "I'm not going to do that."

If you are going to do it, set a time. If you can't set a time, don't do it.

When I first met Peter, it seemed as if he were carrying the weight of the world around with him. Who could have emotional energy in a situation like that? But look at what he did.

Peter, 51: "One of the last things that happened was that my wife said she was going to leave me if I didn't stop worrying about everything all the time. Now I had one more thing to worry about. I know it makes me sound ridiculous, but I was worried about the economy. I was worried about the planet. I was worried about cancer. I was worried about losing money in the stock market. I was worried about my kids because if God wanted to make them not so bright, why did he have to make them lazy too? My father's got dementia, and I was worried about him and my mother.

"But none of that was the biggest thing. It wasn't any one worry. It was the way they added up. That's what drained my energy. That was the biggest thing. Without realizing it, I'd been carrying around an exhausting load of unfinished business.

"It was kind of an accident that turned things around for me. It's funny how it happened. My doctor had told me that I needed to schedule all of these medical tests, routine cancer screening things for a guy my age, like a colonoscopy. Of course I put it off. I was too worried. And so of course it was just one more thing hovering over my life and draining my energy. Suddenly I get this appointment slip from the hospital. It turns out my doctor had just scheduled me in for the first available appointment. [Here it was his doctor who took an item off Peter's to-do list and put it in his appointment book.] I'd been putting it off, and now that I had the appointment, I was relieved. I was finally going to tackle this.

"That night there was a parent-teacher conference for one of my kids, and my wife couldn't go, and I really talked to the teacher. She said, 'Your kid isn't a barn burner, but there's nothing wrong with him either. Just let it go. Stop having such high expectations. You're never going to make him better than he is, so let him be happy being as good as he is.' [Here his kid's teacher took 'worry about your kid's school performance' off Peter's to-do list and threw it in the wastepaper basket.]

"Bang—that got through to me. This was something I didn't have to deal with, like when you get an envelope in the mail and you have that tiny surge of freedom because you throw it away without even opening it.

"I guess that started something. I started dealing with things. Or just taking them off my to-do list. *Fix it or forget it*—that was my new motto.

"It's funny that nothing I did really addressed my worrying directly. I just unhooked myself from unfinished business. But it was almost as if that's what I'd really been worrying about. Not how things would turn out in the world, but about my not dealing with them right. All I know is that once I started either tackling this stuff or letting it go, my worries stopped."

Special Issue:

Emotional Energy and Your Romantic Relationship

Love. But why? Really, what's the point of love? Many of us have never asked this question. And I'm afraid to say I have a very controversial answer.

Romantic love exists for the sake of your emotional energy. That's why we seek love—because it gives us an emotional energy high. Think about the last time you were madly in love. On a scale of one to ten, your energy was . . . eleven? Something like that.

This is a pretty radical thing to say. We're used to saying that love makes the world go round. But we now know that it's energy that makes the world go round. It's love that gives energy a really good push.

Okay. But wait a minute. I left something out. *Good* love produces enormous emotional energy. *Bad* love produces emotional exhaustion. And just the way good love is the most powerful promoter of emotional energy, bad love is the most toxic producer of emotional fatigue.

If we all understood this, it would change our lives. Because right now we've got it backward. We chase love and cling to it because we mistakenly think that love is good in and of itself. But think about what that means. It means we put up with huge amounts of bad love because we think that any love is better than none. And what happens then to our emotional energy? It goes down the tubes, and it's sucked down there by bad love.

But all this is good news for us. If you focus on your emotional energy, then you'll have both more emotional energy and more good love. And how do you do that?

You refuse to put up with bad love.

Think of it like food. Good food can make you feel great. Bad food makes you feel lousy, if it doesn't kill you. So what do you do? Do you eat just so you can say you've eaten? Or do you eat to feel good? Of course you eat to feel good. You don't put up with bad food just because it's food.

So why would you put up with bad love just because in some warped sense it's still called love?

What you need is to be strong enough and filled with enough emotional energy so that you can refuse to put up with bad love in your romantic relationship. It's like going out to dinner. If you're ravenous, you might put up with eating at the first restaurant you can find, even if it serves mediocre food. But if you don't feel desperate to eat, you can hold out for a restaurant that serves great food and makes you feel good for eating there.

So to make it possible for you to say no to bad love in your romantic relationship, bring good love into your life in all your other relationships. The more good love, the better. Nothing will give you more emotional energy faster. It can be love for animals. It can be love for the disadvantaged. It can be love for friends and family. It can be love for whatever you care about. All that matters is that you're actively involved, that it's more than just words, that it gets expressed in things you do.

Then if the romantic love in your life is bad, fix it or move on. Think of bad love as a leaky gas stove. You're not going to live with a gas leak. You're going to fix that stove fast or throw it away. Well, it's the same with love. Not having romantic love is better for you than living with bad love. And you do all this not for the sake of love but for the sake of your energy.

Now let's look at some particular issues that come up for people around their love lives and emotional energy.

Loneliness. When you feel lonely, it hurts your emotional energy. That's one danger. But when you feel lonely, you're likely to settle for bad love. That will hurt your emotional energy even more. And that's an even bigger danger. So what do you do?

If you're on your own, think of it as a time to focus on your relationship with yourself. Discover what you enjoy. Discover how you want to live. Discover what you need. Know who you are above and beyond any relationship you might be in. Build a life that fits who you are. And more than anything, learn to like yourself.

Lynn, 36: "I'd been in this bad marriage for a long time. It wasn't like he was abusing me. It was more that I was with someone who was cold and distant and much too critical. So why did I stay? Why do any of us stay? I made excuses. We all say the same thing. He's really a good guy. I really do love him in spite of everything. But the fact is, I was afraid of being lonely. That's how he held on to me.

"Then one day I was talking to a friend and she said, 'It sounds like you're really lonely with Bob.' Wow, that just hit me. What I was so afraid of, I was already living. I was lonely in this relationship. I didn't look forward to being with him. And most of the time when I was with him it felt awful. The relationship was bringing me down.

"So finally I ended it. Finally. I never felt better in my life. Once I was on my own again, I never had time to be lonely. I was too busy doing things I liked doing. This is going to sound weird, but I was a much better date for myself than Bob ever was for me."

I have an almost mystical belief about this. *The more you learn to like yourself and your life, the faster you'll attract good love.* This means that when you're feeling lonely, instead of filling the void with a stranger while you're in a vulnerable state, take care of yourself, become less vulnerable, and know that this is the way to find love that's good for you.

Conflict. There are two hard questions you have to ask yourself about conflict in your relationship. First, if some issue comes up, would you expect that you and your partner would be likely to end up in conflict? Second, if you did have a conflict with your partner, would you expect that you'd most likely be left feeling bruised?

If you answered yes to either of these questions, there's too much conflict in your relationship and it's doing a number on your energy. It's not really a relationship at all. It's a bad neighborhood filled with dark alleys, and you keep getting mugged. You can't live in a neighborhood like that.

So first you have to see that it can no longer be business as usual. You have to say to yourself, "This level of conflict is killing my energy."

The next thing you have to do is be honest with yourself. There are two explanations for conflict. Either the two of you just can't meet each other's needs or you haven't yet figured out a way to communicate your needs without conflict. Which is it?

You say, "I don't know"? I don't believe you. Of course you know. You're just afraid to admit it. So come on. Face facts. Good love doesn't mean people are able to perfectly meet each other's needs. But if too many needs can't be met too often, good love won't be possible.

Sometimes you just know that your partner doesn't feel right to you. Sometimes it's obvious that the ways the two of you want to live your lives are so divergent that you can't bridge the differences. But the easiest way is for you to think about what your top needs are and then ask yourself how many of them your partner can do a halfway good job of meeting.

Where do you draw the line? First, people rarely change very much. What you see is what you've got. Draw the line wherever you want, but you need to know that if your partner can't meet your important needs, the conflict between you is likely rooted in a problem that can't be fixed.

If you're still not sure, read my book on how to figure out whether you and your partner should stay together. It's called *Too Good to Leave,*

Too Bad to Stay, and it will give you absolutely clear indications about whether there's a basis for your relationship or not.

If you can't meet each other's important needs, you've got to make plans to end the relationship. Otherwise you'll never have anything other than a drain on your emotional energy.

If you can meet each other's needs, you must learn to be more flexible. Make a commitment to achieve greater flexibility for the sake of more emotional energy. Stop fighting over little things. Give yourself time to make decisions together—never feel pressured to make an important decision. Don't be so much in each other's face. Say yes more often. Work at communicating your needs without conflict. *Stop talking about the past, who did what to whom.* Focus on what you want now.

Then read a good couples book, that shows you how to fix your relationship. Or invest in some couples therapy. If you can meet each other's needs, then conflict is not only tragic, it's stupid.

The key to maintaining your emotional energy when you're dealing with relationship issues is to refuse to settle for crappy love. You can make excuses all you want. But from the point of view of energy, if it's not good love, it's bad love. Fix it or let it go. The one thing not to do is stay stuck.

18

It Can Pay to Splurge

Emotional Energy Booster #18

Most people feel deprived. Even spoiled shopaholics. It's not rational. But we have the sense that we give and we give and we give, and what we ultimately get back too often doesn't begin to touch what we feel we really need. So many of us deep down sense that we may go to our graves never having gotten some of the things we've most wanted.

So what if that's not rational? It is how we feel. And it has deep implications for our energy. When you don't get back what you put out, that's a recipe for emotional exhaustion.

⚙

> ## *Diagnostic Question #18*
>
> *Do you have an undercurrent of feeling deprived a lot of the time?*
>
> *A* **yes** *answer to this question means that this secret will give you a big boost of emotional energy.*

Meaningful Splurges

You have to cut at the root of your sense of deprivation. The only way to do so is to splurge on yourself. But it has to be a meaningful splurge. Garden-variety shopping binges just don't cut it.

It's not about indulgence. It's certainly not about spending more money than you can afford. (Whatever you do, don't spend more than you can afford; debt drains emotional energy.) Instead, a meaningful splurge is about doing something that changes how you feel about your life in some small way. It's about setting up a future that makes you feel less deprived.

This is something that compulsive, repetitive shopaholism can't do. A guy who's always buying himself a new tool, a woman who's always buying herself new clothes or jewelry—people like this are doing nothing to end their feelings of deprivation. In fact, they're maintaining them. They're addicted. Needing to have something new leads to only one thing: the need to have something still newer. A moment of satisfaction today leads to more feelings of deprivation tomorrow.

A truly meaningful splurge has got to be on a whole new level. It's got to be the *kind* of thing you'd never give to yourself, a once-in-a-lifetime splurge you will almost certainly not repeat. You're not going to spend more money than you ever spent before. Maybe you'll spend less than you usually spend. But you'll spend your money on something that gives you a big hit of emotional energy.

A meaningful splurge is a gift that keeps on giving. You might be surprised at what falls into this category.

Matt, 41: "I'd always had asthma, but it was pretty mild and I never thought much about it. So when I had a huge asthma attack and had to go to the emergency room, it came as a big shock. I just couldn't breathe. If I hadn't gotten help, I'd have died. Something like that does something to you, believe me. Afterward I was put on medication and the doctors said I should be fine, but I'm thinking I could still die at any minute. I'd never thought that before. It really got me down. I just stopped caring. I had the sense that nothing matters. I went to work every day, but I had to push myself.

"I came home one night when my wife and kids were out of the house. It had been a long time since I was all alone in the house. I looked around and I realized that it just didn't feel like my own house. My wife had done all the decorating. She has good taste, and she consulted me about everything. But it was her show. It was like I was living in a hotel.

"I got mad. I thought maybe I'm going to die, but I don't want to die living in some house that feels strange and alien to me. I wanted to die at home. Yeah, I had a room they called my office. But it was really just filled with junk and papers. And I never spent any time there anyway. So I got this crazy idea in my head that I'd go out and buy some living room furniture and pictures and stuff that I really liked. Chairs that were really comfortable. Couches you could put your feet on. Paintings of the Wild West.

"I thought my wife would have a fit from what I was suggesting, but she just gulped and looked scared and said okay. I told her what I wanted to get rid of and she mostly went along with it. We went to a couple of furniture stores and she mostly let me buy whatever I wanted. 'We'll call our new style eclectic post–asthma-attack,' she said.

"In a way all I did was buy some new living room furniture. But it was amazing how good I felt. It gave me such a boost to hang out in my own living room with furniture that looked right and felt right to me. Somehow it just changed the equation for me. I sort of let go of a sense of doom. Normal life began again for me."

This is a beautiful example of a meaningful splurge. It has nothing to do with spending lots of money. It has everything to do with spending money on something that gives you more satisfaction than you've gotten before.

For example, a lot of women start to feel down when they enter menopause, both from the direct effects of changes in the body and because of what menopause means to them—fears around aging, loss of fertility, loss of beauty, loss of sexuality, and other concerns. One woman who was feeling this way splurged on singing lessons. Twice a week she met with a highly respected singing teacher who was on a university faculty. This was a serious splurge for her. But it was a unique event in her life. Facing what some would think is a real loss, she was giving herself something to replace that loss. The thought of a future filled with beautiful singing canceled out this woman's sense of deprivation.

Another woman had been the manager of an independent bookstore for a number of years and was starting to feel stuck. There was nothing wrong with her life, but she didn't feel she had much of a future to look forward to. Then she did something strange that had a wonderful impact on her energy. She'd been thinking about her father. He'd died a few years earlier, and she missed him terribly. He was a fun, forward-looking guy. And that was the part of her life that was not happening for her, being fun and forward-looking. So she took a couple of her favorite photographs of him and went to someone who painted a portrait of him from the photographs. It was a large portrait she could hang in her living room.

That was a meaningful splurge. Somehow, by doing something big to commemorate what was best in her past, she gave herself the sense that her future would be okay and there'd be good things in it for her.

That's what a meaningful splurge does. I've seen it work with countless people and I've done it myself. I splurged on a new bike, which is, believe me, not the kind of thing I would ever spend money on. I hadn't ridden a bike in thirty years. But I'd wanted to get out more, get more exercise, feel like a kid again, have a new kind of fun. When I was ten, riding my bike all over New York City was my favorite thing to do.

Now I have a new bike again. It gives me just that much of a new and different sense of a future. And I feel a big pickup in my emotional energy.

Emotional energy booster #18
Spend some money on yourself in a way that makes you happy and hopeful.

So let go of your inhibitions and your habits and your old small ways of thinking. Forget about your compulsive, routine buying patterns from the past. Splurge on something meaningful that will give you a new sense of your future.

19

Do Less

Emotional Energy Booster #19

Think about all the different things you did this past week. *How many of them were things you really wanted to do?*

This is a fast route to emotional exhaustion. Your boss asked if you'd work late. A friend asked you to help her out with something. Your mom had something she needed you to do. On Saturday night there was a social get-together that you rather dreaded.

And in case after case, you wanted to say no but you said yes.

Every time you say yes when you want to say no, you end up stressed out, resentful, and a little bit lost, and you have a sense that that you're missing out on things you really need for yourself.

Diagnostic Question #19

Do you do most things because someone else has asked you to do them?

*A **yes** answer to this question means that this secret will give you a big boost of emotional energy.*

A Dirty Little Energy Secret

Here's a dirty little secret about people who have plenty of energy, who accomplish wonderful things and feel so alive. People with emotional energy remember to *just say no*.

They say no to social engagements that other people mindlessly fall into. They say no to their boss sometimes. No to a friend. No to a parent. Sometimes, shocking as it may seem, they say no to a child.

Horrible, you think. Reprehensible.

But I say these people are being smart. We only have so much energy, you and I. When we clutter up our lives with things we have to do that we don't want to do, then we exhaust ourselves. Maybe not today, but tomorrow there will be a price to pay in the form of resentment, fatigue, loss of interest, depression, and loss of a sense of self.

You hear people talking about simplifying their lives. Well, if you *really* want to get a big pop of energy, don't quit your job, sell your house, and move to the country to live on asparagus and wheat you've grown yourself. Instead, say no every once in a while, just for the heck of it, just to feel your own power. Every time you say no, you'll find you've given yourself new options, and you'll find you have a whole new sense of your ability to take care of yourself.

What's So Hard About Saying No?

If saying no is such a great idea, why don't more of us do it? We don't want people to think we're selfish. We're afraid they'll say no back to us. We don't want to be called irresponsible.

Nancy, 29: "My father died when I was little, and my mother had to raise me and my younger brother all by herself. She was a secretary in a law office, and she often had to work late. So I had a lot of responsibility for the house and for taking care of my brother. The truth is, I was a kind of dreamy goofball as a kid. I just wanted to play and hang out and fool around. I didn't want to do things like shop for food and prepare dinner and make sure my brother wasn't getting into trouble.

"As you can imagine, we had a lot of fights, my mother and me. I know she thinks I gave her a lot of trouble, but I think she always won. Ultimately I always did what she wanted me to do. And the *way* she'd always win was by pulling out her big weapon. She'd call me selfish. No, she'd *accuse* me of being selfish. The *very fact* that I was giving her any trouble at all, that I was even hinting at the possibility of wanting to play instead of clean the house, was a sign that there was a stain on my soul. I was a *selfish person*. So of course I was doomed.

"Even if I gave her some lip, the dread of having that stain on my soul was just too much. It was worse than being bad. There was a kind of devil-may-care quality to being bad. Like you were just fun-loving. But being selfish meant you were creepy, dark, and small—evil in a sneaky way. The implication was very clear: If you're selfish, no one will want you. I didn't want no one to want me—it was just the opposite, I desperately wanted to be loved. So at some point I'd start crying almost hysterically, begging my mother to let me help her so I could wipe out the stain.

"Since I've become a grown-up, I've talked to a lot of women about being called selfish. I can't say we've all gotten hit with this, but most of us have, including women who had a father and a mother, plenty of money, and no siblings. It's like one of the two ultimate ways of controlling women. Just tell a woman she's fat or she's selfish, and she'll run screaming from the room, ready to do anything to turn things around.

"This means you say yes a lot. You have a boyfriend and he wants to take a job halfway across the country. Will you come with him? Yes! After all, you're not selfish. And there are all of these things he wants you to do to help him with his life and his career—like wash his shirts or something—because it's too much for him and he'll have a nervous breakdown if he has to deal with it. If you don't do it, you're being selfish.

"It's endless. So we say yes to others. We never say yes to ourselves. We run around like nuts. Overcommitted. Way too busy. And then when we feel really deprived we make everyone pay by going for some extravagant indulgence that's sort of more than we need but not enough of what we really need. And we end up feeling guilty for being selfish anyway.

"I don't think we're going to change. Frankly, I still think women are going to be pretty easy to control by calling them selfish. But I found you don't have to go over to the other side to crawl out from under the burdens.

"*You just have to make a commitment to say no every once in a while, and then you have to really do it.* Once a day, once a week, maybe to your boss, maybe to your friend—maybe even to your mother, God help me—you say no when you could've said yes. You say no to lighten your load. And you say no to give yourself the sense of freedom that comes from knowing you really can say no, and screw them if they don't like it.

"It gets easier as time goes by. The first no is always the hardest. Based on my own experience, once you've said no half a dozen times where you wouldn't have said no before, there's suddenly nothing to it."

You know those poor birds that get covered with oil when there's an oil spill and they can't fly? That's what you feel like when you can't say no. But every time you say no to someone, it's like you've gotten a cleansing bath. You feel light and free.

Raymond, 36: "I'm not going to say it's a sin to be ambitious. Come on. This country was built by ambitious people. You want to get ahead. You want to do things for your family. So you work hard. So what?

"That was the route I took. I said yes to everything. Whatever my boss wanted done, I was the guy ready to do it. If one of the kids' teams needed a coach, I was your man. If my wife wanted me to do something at our church to help out, yeah, sign me up.

"I was just go, go, go. I'd come home and go right to bed. If I had an hour to myself early on a Sunday morning, that was a big deal. But I thought of it as being responsible. A guy would ask me how I found time to do stuff, and I'd say you've got to do what you've got to do.

"From my weird perspective, I was doing everything right, but it was killing me. I got chest pains, and the doctor said it was my heart and that it was because of stress. I'd have to cut back.

"I nearly had a heart attack just thinking about cutting back. You know how some people are pack rats—it would kill them to throw something away? It was like I was a pack rat with my life. Like it would kill me to not do something. But that's what was killing me. All the things I was doing.

"My doctor put it to me this way: 'If you die, where will your family be?' He was speaking my language. That's been my whole thing, being responsible. But I was getting it all wrong. Running around piling stuff on my plate like a crazy man at a buffet is not being responsible. Being afraid to say no is not being responsible.

"First of all, I'm entitled to enjoy my life. What if I die and go to heaven and the first thing God says to me is 'This gift of life I gave you, did you enjoy it?' What am I going to say: 'Sorry, God, but I was too busy to enjoy Your precious gift'? No, I have a responsibility to get more out of my life than I've been getting.

"The other thing is that by saying yes to everything and really doing too much, there's no focus in my life. It's kind of bizarre. I'm ambitious, so I do all this stuff, and then I piss away my ambition with a bunch of stuff that doesn't add up to anything. Whom am I helping?

"So I said to myself, 'That's it—there's going to be a lot more of me saying no around here.'

"I thought there'd be this big crisis in my family when I started saying no to some of the things they asked me to do. Like some school function where you don't really need both parents to show up. It was kind of humbling, but no one really noticed. What they did notice, many weeks later, was that I seemed a lot happier. My wife and one of my sons said that now when I was with them, it was like I really wanted to be with them. I guess that's what it means to have emotional energy in your life. When you're there, you're really there.

"And the way to do that is to say no sometimes."

Emotional energy booster #19
Stop doing things you don't want to do.

There are always ways you can stop doing what you don't want to do, even if you just cut down a little. You don't have to turn your life upside down or become a different person. It has nothing to do with completely changing your priorities or your lifestyle. All that's exhausting in itself.

What you do have to do is a lot easier. Just cut back. Just stop doing *some* things you don't want to do. Say no here and there. Part of this is about simplifying and de-stressing your life. But a big part of it is getting the sense of empowerment that comes from knowing you can say no.

When you know you can say no, then and only then do you know that you're free. And there's nothing better than a sense of freedom to give you more emotional energy.

20

Go to Confession

Emotional Energy Booster #20

Here I am, a Jew, telling you to go to confession. What's up with that?

Of course, I'm not talking just about confessing to a priest. Besides, my job is to tell the truth about emotional energy. They say confession is good for the soul. Well, it's just as good for your emotional self. Guilt is stupid in any case, but even if you're not feeling guilty, confession is still a powerful and straightforward way to give yourself more emotional energy.

Powerful Medicine, Handle Carefully

Before we go any further, I have to warn you. Confessions can be wonderful medicine, but they're also very powerful and can be dangerous if used in the wrong way. *You should only confess to someone who can offer you understanding and forgiveness. And you should only confess to someone who won't be hurt by your confession.*

Let's say you cheated on your spouse or hurt your best friend in business. You might think you'll feel better if you confess to the person you betrayed. But it's guaranteed that you'll make the other person feel far worse. The thing you're doing to unburden yourself is *giving* the other person an even bigger burden. He or she will lose far more emotional energy than you'll gain. There will be anger and hurt and distance between you. Any temporary gain in emotional energy will quickly turn to loss.

There's a simple way to guarantee you're confessing the right thing to the right person. Just ask yourself, "Will the other person feel that he or she is hearing bad news?" If you honestly answer yes, then this is the wrong confession to make to this particular person. That's the warning. But if you make your confession to someone who can handle it, who won't think it's bad news, you'll have a rush of emotional energy that will last a long time.

The Beauty of Confession

Diagnostic Question #20

Do you feel burdened by guilt? Do you feel you've done something terrible you want to get off your chest?

A **yes** *answer to either of these questions means that this secret will give you a big boost of emotional energy.*

Twenty-five years ago I learned from my friend Jenny just how important confession can be as a way to lift oneself out of emotional exhaustion. You have to understand that I had a blind spot when it came to this issue.

First of all, I can never hold anything back from anybody. I literally cannot look in the face of anyone I care about if I haven't told them about something I might've done that they have a right to know. I've always been this way. That and a shamefully boring life have given me few opportunities to unburden myself by confessing.

Second, as a psychotherapist, I hear people confess things to me every day. And that made it hard for me to see how special confession is as a source of emotional energy. I couldn't see it because it was right under my nose.

That's when Jenny opened my eyes. She was a colleague whose background was similar to mine, and we were getting together to talk about writing a paper about the psychological impact of being a child of Holocaust survivors. She was a bright, talkative woman, a few years older than me. This was going to be one of the first papers either of us had ever written.

I was disappointed when I found that she had little to offer. It felt as if she were holding back, but it didn't make any sense that she would do that. Now let Jenny pick up the story as she wrote it twenty-five years ago.

Jenny, 31 (at the time): "I think what hung me up was the fact that for me the Holocaust was an almost sacred event. Everyone in my family except for my actual parents was killed in the Holocaust. So I think I must've felt you had to be clean somehow to touch it. All I know is that when I started working with Mira on that paper I went into a fog, like someone who hasn't slept in three days. I just wasn't myself. It was something I really wanted to do, and yet I wasn't showing up for it at all.

"At the same time I was starting to obsess about something I'm still very ashamed of. Back when I was in college I was basically the school slut. Guys would tell other guys that if you want a guaranteed lay, just ask Jenny out. Jenny the Joy Girl. Almost everyone who took me out got lucky on the first date. I mean, I hated this about myself, and I tried to fight it. I'd go for a couple of months without going out with anybody, but then I'd start sleeping around again. I felt very lonely and powerless and unattractive. I thought I was a nothing, basically. So I got in a trap. I'd sleep with guys to feel like somebody. Sex gave me power. But being a slut eventually made me feel like I was nothing again. And the only way I knew to feel like a somebody was to sleep with somebody. I was trapped in a cycle.

"I got out of it, thank God. Practically the first guy I met in graduate school—it was a new town, and I'd done nothing to give myself a reputation—really liked me, and we fell in love and he kind of saved me from myself. But I never stopped feeling terrible for what I'd done. I felt I was a slut—I still do in a way, even though I haven't acted like that since I got married.

"So there I am working with Mira on what was for me a sacred theme and I'm carrying around this secret that I'm a slut. I felt that if she knew, she wouldn't want to work with me. Or she would, but she'd secretly feel I was really screwed up. But I saw how I was messing up, acting like someone who had nothing to contribute. And I knew I was obsessing about my past.

"I got to the point where I felt I had nothing to lose. So one Friday morning we met for coffee in this out-of-the-way place—it was to talk about our paper—and I confessed my sins. Just the way Catholics confess to their priests. I practically said, 'Mira, forgive me, for I have sinned.' I told her story after story of these guys who really used me and how I let them use me. And I kept thinking, 'God, what kind of creature does she think I am?'

"But the funny thing is that most of the time people don't care what you've done in the past as long as you didn't do it to them! Mira knew I wasn't a bad person. What did she care what I'd done in the past? In fact, before I felt my own relief I felt how relieved Mira was. She'd known something was making me stupid, but she couldn't figure out what it was. Now she knew why I'd been holding back.

"Of course, I cried a lot, even though we were sitting in a restaurant. But I felt so much relief at getting that off my chest. I'd never told anyone any of it before. Now I'd told her everything. Even my husband still doesn't know anything about how many guys I've slept with. I don't know if he could handle knowing.

"It was amazing how much better I felt right away. I didn't even mind crying in public. But Mira accepted me completely. And then it was as if those bad things I'd done got very small and very far away, like something naughty you did when you were a child that no one cares about. It was like she saw me. The real me. The naked me, as I really was, with all my terrible imperfections, and she loved me anyway. It was as if I didn't have to be afraid in the world anymore. And in fact, in our working together from that point on I opened up. It was like I had permission to be alive."

Jenny has gone on to lead a happy and productive life that brought her much satisfaction. She says today that her confession to me twenty-five years ago marked the turning point. She went from being stuck and lost to being productive and having direction.

It's important to see that everyone, without exception, carries around the guilty knowledge of dark deeds and even darker thoughts. Everyone. Everyone carries around a kind of invisible mud on their shoes, and everyone is secretly afraid of being caught tracking this mud in wherever they go. One of the things people say about themselves more commonly than almost anything else is "I'm afraid that if people really knew me, they wouldn't like me." They are talking about their guilty secrets.

All this makes us feel we're not entitled to getting everything good there is out of life. That's why when you confess you feel a big hit of emotional energy. When you confess, something happens to your guilty secret. It looks smaller than you thought it was. Less evil. More normal. Everything seems scarier in the dark than it does in the light. Plus you're given a chance to do something to make up for what you did. And the other person usually says something reassuring that makes you feel forgiven.

That's why it's so important to pick the right person to confide in. You've got to make it easy for yourself. Confide in a friend. A member of the clergy. A therapist. A doctor. Maybe even a stranger, someone you strike up a conversation with at a lunch place or on a trip. You'll be surprised to find that your confession will most likely elicit a confession from the other person. In the end you'll both feel more alive.

You can confess something besides your own bad deed too. Many of us are just as ashamed, if not more so, of bad things that happened to us.

People who have been sexually or physically abused or threatened have a guilty secret they need to confess. It's not that they did something. But even the things that happened to us make us feel guilty because we feel there must be something wrong with us if this bad thing happened to us in the first place.

Confession frees up all the energy spent hiding and feeling bad.

I know that most of the time we sail through life as if this doesn't matter. But all that says is that a person can learn to adjust to the weight he carries. Fat men can be graceful dancers. But that doesn't mean they don't carry a huge burden. So the fact that you're coping is great, but it doesn't mean your guilty secret isn't a huge burden.

I can prove the benefit of confessing a secret. An amazing social experiment happened over the past forty years. As recently as 1960 almost all gay people kept their sexual orientation hidden. That's when the movement to come out of the closet began. By 1970 it was gathering steam. Between 1980 and 1990 it was roaring along. By now there's a sense that there's something wrong with you if you *hide* the fact that you're gay.

And the evidence is overwhelming. Society had made being gay a guilty secret. "Confessing" this secret to friends, family, coworkers, and others took away the guilt, the fear, the isolation, the sense that there was something wrong with you. It was a way of staking a claim to life, of giving yourself permission to be alive as your true self.

Virtually without exception, gay men and women reported enormous surges in energy when they revealed the truth about themselves. They said that they'd had no idea how much energy they'd used keeping themselves hidden and being afraid of being found out. And this is even more striking when you realize that they often faced hostility and rejection when they revealed who they really were. Still, "confession" was good for the soul.

Emotional energy booster #20
Find someone to confess your darkest secret to.

There is someone in your life who can handle the truth about what you've done or what's been done to you or who you are. This is someone who won't be threatened by your disclosure. You know who this person is. There are probably a number of people like this in your life.

You don't have to make a big deal of this if you don't want to. And it doesn't have to be a big, earth-shattering confession. But the next time you're talking to this person, unburden yourself. You'll have taken a big step toward putting the emotional energy factor at the center of your life.

Special Issue:

Emotional Energy and
Your Work Life

There's a memorable scene in *Snow White and the Seven Dwarfs,* where it's early morning and the dwarfs are headed for a day of labor in their mine. And they sing happily, "Heigh ho, heigh ho, it's off to work we go."

Now, *that's* an image of emotional energy in the workplace. It's what we all want, a situation where we bring emotional energy to our work and in turn our work gives emotional energy back to us.

Unfortunately, most of us don't live in a Disney cartoon. In fact, for many of us work is a major trouble zone. It's boring at best, too often discouraging or humiliating. Two of the worst things that can happen to us when it comes to energy happen in our work lives: We feel trapped and we feel confused. We don't want to be where we are but don't know how to get out, and we don't know where to go and don't know how to get there. And you can't get much energy from spending thirty years dreaming about retirement.

Getting Emotional Energy from Work

At least you know you're not alone. What you may not know is that there are things you can do to change your relationship with your work life. And you know this is true. You know there are people in a situation similar to yours who've either gotten unstuck or who seem to be getting a lot more emotional energy from their work life than you are. What's their secret?

Know where you want to go next. Everyone is trapped. Even the president of the United States is stuck in his job for four years, and he's expected to opt for another four years. So that's not the difference between people who get emotional energy from their work and those who don't. The difference is having a sense of where you want to go next.

People who feel stuck say, "I'm going to be here forever." People with energy say, "Three years from now, here's where I'm going to be. . . ." That's all you need. Just a hint, a taste, a whiff, of the possibility of being somewhere else and at least the vaguest sense of how you're going to get there.

So let me put it to you. Where do you want to go next that you think you have a shot of getting to? Even if you later change your mind, just having something in mind will give you emotional energy.

It doesn't matter what it is. Getting a better job. Getting your boss's job. Learning new skills. Moving into an area where you'll make more money or get to make more decisions. Getting out of the rat race. Owning your own business. Doing something more creative.

All you need is a sense of what you want to do next. Then do what works to make that happen.

You know, ultimately it's we who give ourselves energy. If you do one little thing every week that brings your next step closer, you'll fill yourself with hope because you'll know you're doing things to take care of your future. Think of your future as a baby. You wouldn't starve or neglect a baby. Why would you do the same to your future?

Emphasize the positive. I always ask patients and people I interview to tell me about their best job and their worst job. As you know, there are some pretty bad jobs out there. For yourself, maybe there was the time you had the boss from hell. Maybe there was the time you had to work twenty-eight hours a day. Maybe there was the time you were under terrible pressure to perform and you just didn't know what you were doing. Maybe there was the time you were painfully underpaid for working like a dog.

Well, if you know you're going somewhere better and different in the future, you can do something now that really works to get more energy from your job. And that's to emphasize the positive. Every job has its good points. Are you working on a chain gang? That's not the best of jobs, but at least it's building up your muscles and giving you a chance to lose weight. Just think of the camaraderie. And you get to sing on the job!

You get my point. Once you know you're not trapped, focusing on the good things becomes doable and a shortcut to emotional energy. You have a bad boss? Well, at least you're learning bit by bit to deal with difficult bosses. But maybe you're also being challenged to do a higher level of work. Or maybe you're being given the opportunity to work more on your own. Maybe you're just learning a lot.

So what are the three best things about your current job? They could be things you enjoy, or things you're allowed to get away with, or things that are helping you grow that you can transfer to a better job. Knowing the three best things makes it much easier to see your job in a positive light.

Another way you can approach this is to ask yourself how your current job is an opportunity for . . . what? Every job is an opportunity for something. Maybe it's just an opportunity for reminding yourself that you'll never ever again do this kind of work. But whatever it's an opportunity for, if you focus on it, you'll feel more positive and have more emotional energy.

Have your own agenda. Deep down I think we all know that work is a place where, in exchange for paying you, your boss owns you. It's not polite to emphasize that, and when jobs are plentiful a boss can't push this fact too hard or he'll lose his employees, but this is the basic deal.

So we exist on a job to further the boss's and the company's agendas. Fine. Rationally we can accept that. But emotionally it's hard to take.

The solution is to develop an agenda of your own and to make sure you're furthering it. This doesn't have to be a big deal. Maybe your agenda is to use your current job to enhance your résumé so you can get a better job. Maybe your agenda is to pull down a paycheck so you can pay the rent until you find a way to change careers. Maybe your agenda is to add to your paper clip collection. (Not that I'm advocating employee theft!) But you get my point. You've got to have something that you're getting for yourself that you can point to that's furthering your goals, your interests.

This goes beyond emphasizing the positive. The positive points of your job are just good things you're getting now. Furthering your own agenda is about using your job to get good things for yourself in the future.

You have to ask yourself what you want. Maybe all you want is to have congenial coworkers. If that's your agenda, admit it, congratulate yourself on having it, and look forward to having more of it in your future.

Lots of people get into trouble because they can't be clear or honest with themselves about what their agenda really is. One woman sold ad time for a ratio station. What she liked about her job was hanging out with people, talking about music, and showing them how to improve their business by advertising. That was her agenda: to get paid for doing that. Unfortunately, many months when the new sales figures were posted she wasn't at the top of the list. And she'd experience terrible discouragement. Her energy took a big hit. But none of this was necessary. Being the top salesman was not her agenda. So why suffer when she was shown up as not being that? *Success on the job isn't about what you accomplish for others, it's about what makes you feel successful for yourself.* If this woman could be honest about her agenda, she'd see she was satisfying it every day. The truth is that she didn't care about being number one.

Whatever your agenda, that's the part of *you* that is actually rewarded by doing the work you do. It's only by knowing your agenda and developing it that you experience these rewards. And that's how you get every last little bit of emotional energy from your work.

21

Feel Good from the Outside In

Emotional Energy Booster #21

Hey, good-looking. I can see you, you know, and you look pretty darn good. But can I be frank? Don't be angry with me, but the fact is that you could look better. You *have* looked better.

And this is surprisingly important for your emotional energy.

Do people look good because they have emotional energy? Or do they have emotional energy because they do things to look good?

Who knows? But I do know this: People with emotional energy look good. People who get more emotional energy look better.

The next time you're at a gathering, see who catches your eye and holds it. Yes, there will be good-looking faces that initially capture your attention. But in many cases your attention drifts. And you find that you're actually more drawn to someone not classically beautiful but who seems to be attractive. What is that something that trumps luscious lips and great bone structure? It's the radiant zest and happiness that come with emotional energy.

Diagnostic Question #21

Are you happy with your appearance? Have you done something meaningful to make yourself look better?

A no *answer to either question means that this secret will give you a big boost of emotional energy.*

Start Looking Better Immediately

Emotional energy booster #21
It doesn't matter where you're starting from or what you do.
But do something that'll make you feel you look better.

You don't have to wait to get emotional energy to start looking better. You can do things to start looking better and you'll get more emotional energy. It's not vanity. It's a psychologically savvy investment in creating an outside that gives you energy on the inside.

This applies to all of us. Whether you're a gorgeous model or you've settled into a frumpy, fraying-around-the-edges middle age, there are an enormous number of things you can do to look better. And the amazing fact is that every single thing you do will give you more emotional energy.

The key is that you have to do something *more* than you've been doing or something *different* from what you've been doing. If you already go to the gym every day or buy a new pair of Manolo Blahniks every week, then another gym day or another pair of shoes isn't going to do it for you. The point is, no more business as usual. Take it up a notch, or go in a different direction.

Look, I'm not a stylist, a makeover specialist, a fitness guru, or a fashion maven. I don't have any earthshaking revelations about things to do to look good. And I certainly don't want to get into controversies—what to do to look better is something people have an amazing number of opinions about. Don't do anything you don't want to do.

I just know that there are countless men and women who made earthshaking changes in their emotional energy by doing things to look good that they would never have thought of doing. And that's the big obstacle. It's not how-to-look-good tips that are in short supply; it's opening our minds to trying things that we might never have let ourselves consider before. Here are a couple of stories. You don't have to agree with what they did for themselves. The important point is doing something big and new and different to make yourself look better.

Matt, 53: "I'd always been a gym rat. I love working out. And I do it right too. I do the aerobics machines and the weights. The whole package. But when I turned fifty, it must be genes because my whole face turned haggard and drooping and tired-looking. It was bizarre. Overnight I went from looking younger than my age to looking older than my age.

"I did what I always do—I worked out harder. But that didn't help, and it really bothered me. The thing is, it happened at the same time I was plateauing at the bank. Maybe I'd never have a shot at the top job. It all made me feel down.

"How many times a day do you think you look in the mirror? One day I counted and I discovered that I took a good look at myself in the mirror at least ten times. A few times in the bathroom in the morning. Every time you go to the washroom at work. Mirrors you pass in the hallway or in your living room. And then your bathroom again at night. Ten times easy. And every time you do, you see this old guy looking at you and it kind of drags you down.

"I think it's always a problem for someone when the way they think they look bums them out. And that was happening to me. I was *there*.

"Plastic surgery had never entered my mind. Yeah, I'm a banker now, but—true confessions—when I was in college I was a hippie, and right afterward too. We hated the very idea of plastic surgery. Only the worst people in the world would do something like that, we thought.

"I don't know how I made the switch. I think I was waiting for my wife one night when we were going out and I was looking through one of her magazines. There was some article about plastic surgery—for women, of course. It was very matter-of-fact, not silly the way you think a woman's magazine is going to be. And it hit me. I can do that. Why the hell not?

"And I did. I went for the face-lift. Facial liposuction. Eyelids. The works. I felt self-conscious, like it wasn't something I was supposed to do. But afterward, when all the swelling and discoloration went away, I felt like a million bucks. It was such a boost. It was like I had a secret weapon. And when I went back to work I knew I looked a lot better, and everyone else thought so too. It was like I'd come back to work after winning an award. I'm a big fan of plastic surgery now. If you think it might be right for you, check it out, and if it makes sense, do it. You won't believe how great you'll feel."

Meg, 39: "Was it turning 39? I don't know. But I started hating the way I looked. I felt bored with my appearance. And I think I just felt bored in general. It was all very confusing because I spent a lot of money on clothes, and at the same time I felt that women who lived to shop were very shallow. I'm one of the curators at a local museum. We're a funny combination of scholars and administrators. It's not like I run an art gallery. People like me aren't supposed to live for how they look.

"I have these expensive suits and dresses that I hate. It's like I dressed to show rich people I was solid myself. But it just made me look boring. You know sometimes you reach the point where you can't take it any-more? I felt so bad about myself. This was hard because women always say they have nothing to wear. But I decided I had to have a whole new look. I decided to throw everything away and start fresh.

"I spoke to a couple of image consultants until I found someone who understood how radical I wanted to go but who also had a clue about what kind of person I was. And we came up with this concept for a hip, young, downtown New York kind of look, where you combine fun boutique kinds of clothes with cool, classic items from vintage clothing stores. It was a very unique look that made me feel special.

"But it was a total fashion transformation, like jeans or velvet pants instead of tweed skirts. Every time I saw myself in the mirror I felt great, fantastic. My new look gave me enormous confidence. All those people I'd been afraid of—now it was like I was daring them to criticize me, but they couldn't because I looked so fine. I felt so happy."

Plastic surgery. Fashion makeovers. These are just two ideas for looking better than you do already. Certainly you don't have to do either of these things. And certainly the social pressure to look great shouldn't run your life. The best thing is to accept yourself the way you are.

Still, we have to face facts. And it's a fact that people get emotional energy when they feel they look good, and they get more emotional energy when they feel they look better. It's not about how other people make you feel. It's about how you feel for yourself.

Do whatever makes sense to you, whatever feels right to you. Maybe you should dress up more often. Maybe you should schedule a night out once a month where you dress to the hilt and go out on the town. Maybe you're self-conscious about your smile. It's never too late to get your teeth whitened or straightened. The more emotional energy you get, the more you smile. And the more you smile, the more you'll get emotional energy. Sign up with a personal trainer—good ones work wonders.

It doesn't matter what you do. It matters that you do something more than you've been doing, or something different. The point is, take a leap and do something fresh to look better.

22

Never Let Yourself
Feel Pressured

Emotional Energy Booster #22

Suppose you have to explain to someone how to do something that you know how to do very well. It's easy. Now suppose you have to explain how to do that thing on TV in front of millions. That's pressure. Suppose while you're talking someone's yelling at you to hurry up before you're cut off. That's pressure. Suppose someone's life depends on whether you can perfectly explain how to do this thing. That's pressure.

Feeling under pressure is a major source of emotional exhaustion. Just think about what happens to children who are overpressured by adults. They shrink and cower within themselves, and ultimately they collapse in one way or another. This has happened, for example, to many budding young tennis stars who had too much pressure put on them. They weren't necessarily working harder physically than other up-and-coming players, but they were under much more emotional pressure. And in almost every case their zest for the game, their resilience, and their ability to function were damaged.

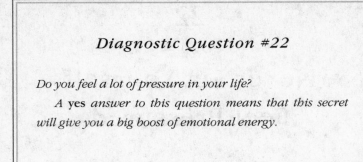

Diagnostic Question #22

Do you feel a lot of pressure in your life?
*A **yes** answer to this question means that this secret will give you a big boost of emotional energy.*

A Shortcut to Pressure-free Living

It's possible to reduce the pressure you're living under. "How can that be?" you might ask. "I mean, people put pressure on me all the time, and I have to respond, don't I?"

Here's the trick. Yes, there's pressure everywhere. Yes, sometimes there's nothing you can do about it. But there are places in your life where you *can*. And every time you do something somewhere to reduce the pressure on you, it will give you more emotional energy. Then you'll be able to cope better in those situations where there's nothing you can do about it.

I know you have it in you to avoid being affected by the pressure someone tries to apply to you. For example, when a telemarketer calls you to try to get you to buy something, I'm sure you say no lots of times. Well, then, there you are. You've just proven that you can resist pressure. Now all you have to do is apply your proven resistance to the 101 situations that crop up in your life where up until now you have felt pressured.

And I'll show you exactly how to do this. I promise you a little miracle. You will be able in a surprising number of cases to stop feeling pressured. And because of this you will feel an amazing rebound of energy.

Perhaps the best way to show you how to do this is to tell you about two people and show you what they did.

George, 42: "I'll admit that I had a difficult past, to put it mildly. I dropped out of school, and I got into a lot of trouble with drugs and alcohol. I was behind the eight ball in my life. I was going down the tubes. By some kind of miracle I got involved in this program to help men turn their lives around. We got computer training, training on how to function on the job, all kinds of help to allow us to function like normal people.

"Then I started my first job, and right away I started feeling I was in trouble. I'm not saying my boss was a bad guy. But he was a tough guy. He'd ask you a question and it was like he was pointing a knife at your gut. Or he'd come up to the computer where you were working and he'd ask you to do something while he was standing over you. And it was like he'd poked a gun in your side. He'd say, 'Do this now' or 'Give me the answer now.' And whatever smarts I had, the pressure made me stupid.

"Man, I'd get so nervous. I'd sweat. And feel weak. All that pressure. I just couldn't take it.

"In the past I'd have walked off. Of course, that's how I'd ruined my life. But what else was I going to do? I knew I was in big trouble. So I went to see one of the counselors in our program. Man, he really helped me.

"He said, 'Wait a minute. You're putting all this on your boss. Like he's the only one with any power here. Yeah, he's your boss, so he asks you questions and he asks you to do things. So what? But it's you who's turning it into a whole big pressure thing. You're the one letting the pressure get to you.'

"So he told me what to do. First he said, 'Look, just because he's asking you a question doesn't mean you have to answer right then and there. And it doesn't mean your answer has to be perfect. Take the pressure off yourself. Buy time for yourself. Tell him you'll get back to him by the end of the day, or by the end of the week, or by Monday, or whatever. Feel free to say you don't know, you'll have to work on it. You can say you've got a rough guess but you'll have to give it some more thought. The point is that you don't have to assume there's pressure if there isn't any.

"'But here's the other thing. Suppose he *is* putting pressure on you. Suppose he *does* want you to answer right away or turn out something perfect. He's boss of you, but he's not boss of the universe. You can say you can't give him the answer right now, that you know he wants you to answer right away, but is there any reason this can't wait a little? Or you can say you know he needs you to do this just right, but you can't do it just right. All you can do is your best at this point.

"'Here's the deal. He puts the pressure on. Okay. But you politely take the pressure off. The point is, you don't have to buy into it. You don't have to get stampeded. You're a worthwhile person. You can have a say in how fast you do things and how good they have to be.'"

This advice saved George's life. He'd always had a hard time dealing with pressure, but so do most of us. And it's devastating to our emotional energy. The fear and pain in life become enormous. But as George showed, there are two simple things you can do to turn a pressure situation into one that gives you emotional energy.

First, don't assume that anyone's putting pressure on you. Maybe someone's asking you to do something, but who says you're being asked to do it right away? Who says you have to do it just right? Maybe not. You can check it out. Or you can do it at your own pace and in your own way and see if that's all right.

Second, even if you are having pressure put on you, who says you have to go along with it? Maybe they're saying you have to do it now. Why can't you say "Let me do it later"? Maybe they're saying you've got to do a wonderful job. Why can't you say "Let me do the best job I can"?

But what if the pressure *really* is on? What if there really is a demand that you work fast and do it just right? Are you screwed? Are you doomed to emotional exhaustion? No. You still have some power. You don't always have to succumb by feeling pressured. Liz illustrates this.

Liz, 28: "Right now I'm the top salesman for the top rock-and-roll radio station in a major city. Not bad for someone my age. Frankly, I have a good personality for sales. Who I am works in this business. But there's a part of me that almost killed me. When I was starting out I'd let the pressure get to me. I'd push too hard. I'd panic if I felt I was going to lose a sale. I'd get pushy and overbearing. And then I'd sort of collapse. When the pressure was put on me I went right along with it and put more pressure on myself.

"What saved me was playing tennis. I loved playing tennis, but I was far from being the best player in the world. I'd run around the court like a nut, getting wild, losing control. Flailing at the ball. Overrunning it. Hitting wild shots. I was very erratic.

"I play regularly with this older guy. I'm younger and faster than he is. I probably have more basic athletic ability. But he beats me pretty consistently. And that bugged the hell out of me. I should be a better player, but I'm running around like a nut and he's winning.

"At one point I asked him what his secret was, because I was so jealous. He asked if it would be all right if he criticized me a little. I said sure. And he said that he'd noticed that if he just puts a little pressure on me, I blow up and get wild. He said he used to be like that but that he'd learned to do something much better. He said he learned that there's a big difference between feeling pressure and losing control.

"'Okay, so I've hit the ball to you down the line at a pretty good pace,' he told me. 'You feel pressure. You've got to really struggle to get to the ball. But who said you have to get wild? Who said you can't decide to play a controlled game and play within yourself? Yeah, you run to the ball, but you don't go nuts. You swing at the ball, but you still take a nice controlled swing. Maybe you'll lose the point anyway. But here's the thing. If I beat you, I beat you. That was me doing it. My shot was too good. These things happen. But you never beat yourself. You're in control of yourself. You're hitting a smooth, safe, smart shot.'

"That was what turned it all around for me. It was the idea that even when you really are under pressure you should never beat yourself. If on a sales call the other guy's giving you a hard time, okay, maybe you're going to lose this one. But you're going to talk to the guy in a good way. You're just not going to let the pressure get to you. Even if you have to respond quickly, even if you have to come up with something brilliant, you're going to stay cool, and relax, and know that you're doing your best.

"Suppose someone puts a gun to your head and says he's going to blow your brains out unless you tell him what the capital of Montana is. Sure, it's natural to panic. But if you want to save your life, you've got to relax and not feel pressure. Otherwise how the hell can you possibly remember what the capital of Montana is?

"When you're under pressure, all you can do is your best. If your best isn't good enough, what can you possibly do about that? But why let your sense of feeling pressured prevent you from doing your best? That means you're always smart. What I found is that when you focus on doing your best—even if you're afraid that might not be good enough—instead of focusing on how much pressure you're under, you really *do* do your best."

Emotional energy booster #22
Sometimes you really are under pressure. But if you focus
on yourself and try to do your unrattled,
unflappable best, you'll be fine.

Practice Makes Perfect

You're in the supermarket with your kid. She's whining and fussing for you to buy her some particular breakfast cereal. Okay, but just because she's *putting* pressure on you doesn't mean you have to respond by *feeling* pressured. And what you can do with your kid you can do with your boss, your spouse, your parents, your friends, and everyone else who's trying to put pressure on you.

Practice this every chance you get in your everyday life. Every time you feel pressure, *refuse to participate*. That's the ultimate key to getting the pressure off. Maybe you'll find that the pressure's not really there at all. Maybe you don't have to deal with the pressure. But even if the pressure *is* there and you have to deal with it, you can refuse to participate in feeling pressured. Refuse to buy into time pressure, and as for the pressure to be perfect, focus on doing your best. Then you will do your best.

23

Confidence Is a Choice

Emotional Energy Booster #23

In people's lifelong journey to improve themselves, confidence is the Holy Grail. With it, you can walk on water. Without it, you're soggy toast. That's why we all want it. What gives you more emotional energy than confidence, than knowing that you can step up to a challenge and win?

Let's say you're running a marathon. It's near the end. You're exhausted, but no more so than anyone else. And you have a fragile lead. Suddenly another runner makes a move and starts to pass you. You've been struggling to hold on, and he suddenly has this surge of energy.

It's at a moment like this that confidence—being able to say "I can win"—gives you the emotional energy to try a little harder. Otherwise the other runner's surge is like a knife in your heart and you collapse. And we don't have to just focus on runners' marathons. Much of what we do is a marathon of some sort or another—trying to get a promotion at work, bringing up children, saving for the down payment for a house.

We all know how confidence is the difference between getting what you want and not getting it. I knew a young woman—attractive but not stunning—who would go out on the weekends to clubs, confident that she could get any guy she wanted to ask her out. Her friends, deeply impressed, told me how her very confidence gave her a magnetic presence that made men want her.

Then there're the rest of us. We've stepped up to the plate a lot and unfortunately we've struck out a lot. We can look back on mistakes, failures, disasters. In many ways our confidence has had the crap beaten out of it.

Diagnostic Question #23

Do you feel you could do more or be more if only you had more confidence?

A **yes** *answer to this question means that this secret will give you a big boost of emotional energy.*

Loss of confidence is devastating for our emotional energy. Without confidence, the two most horrible words in the English language take hold of us: "Why try?" These words are horrible because they're the beginning of doom for any enterprise we care about, including love.

This brings us right to the trap we get into when we lose confidence. It's important to understand this trap because only when you do can you see a way out. The good news is that this terrible trap is so easy to get out of when you know how. What's sad is that more people don't know how to get out of it.

Breaking Free of the No-Confidence Trap

We base our feelings of confidence on being able to win. But it's tough to win, and we have too many losses. So we lose confidence. Then we either stop trying altogether or we try to win at an easier game. Most people find their level and are content. But the minute they think of playing the tougher game, they have to face their shaken confidence.

It seems like a trap you can't escape. You can't win without confidence. You can't get confidence without winning. Bye-bye, energy.

But this is an illusion.

Here's the truth. And this is the secret of confidence that high-energy people know. If you open your mind and heart to this secret and let it in and act on it, you'll get all the confidence you need. This is what confident people do that anyone can do.

Emotional energy booster #23
The secret of confidence is focusing on what you can control, not on what you can't.

Think about something in your life where you don't feel very confident. Queasy. Weak in the knees. Faint with lack of emotional energy. Ask yourself what's making you so unconfident. Almost certainly it's your thinking about an outcome that you have no control over. Your boss is not going to like your presentation, you think. The person you want to ask out isn't going to want to go out with you. You're not going to meet your sales quota. You're going to perform poorly during the charity golf tournament.

What unconfident people don't understand is that no one in the world could possibly feel confident about situations where the outcome is uncertain if all they focus on is the outcome. It's an iron rule in life. Either the outcome is unlikely—winning the golf tournament, for example—and it's crazy to feel confident you'll win. Or the outcome is likely—making a decent cake from a cake mix, for example—and you haven't really accomplished anything worth feeling confident about. So it *never* makes sense to focus on the outcome when it comes to confidence.

The secret of confident people is that they focus on what they *know* they can do and then they do that in the best way they can. And they don't worry about the outcome. The batter steps up to the plate. All he can do is keep his eye on the ball and do his best. That's what all the good hitters do.

You have to make a presentation to your boss? Don't worry about whether he's ultimately going to approve your plan. If he's in a bad mood or he's been told to make cuts, the outcome is out of your hands. All you can do is what you *know* you can do and then do that in the best way you can. For example, walk into the meeting sure of your facts. Come up with a good argument. Research the competition. Have an idea of what his beliefs and enthusiasms are and be prepared to deal with them. If you prepare like this, you won't have to worry about anything else.

Maybe you're afraid your voice will quiver when you make your presentation. That happens to some people. But if you can't control it, get confidence instead by focusing on what you can control, like having a plan for how you'll deal with it, such as apologizing in advance for being nervous when you present. That way you'll gain sympathy for being so open: You were confident enough in yourself to reveal an imperfection.

Staying in the Moment

In the final motivating minutes before a big game, Hall of Fame pro football coach Marv Levy used to ask one question: "Where do you want to be?" And the players would shout out the required answer: "Right here! Right now!" There was nothing about "We're going to win." It was all about being in the moment, because that's where you can focus on what you can control. If you want to be in the moment, you can control the moment. If you can control the moment, you'll always have confidence.

Here are two people who got a tremendous boost of energy by making a shift from thinking about outcomes that destroyed their confidence to thinking about processes they could control that gave them confidence.

The first is a best-selling writer, and, as always, I've changed his name. But it's important to see how people you'd think of as being very confident have wrestled with the same demons we all have. This is a demon you can wrestle with and win if you know how.

Brian, 48: "Let me tell you a story about me I've never told anyone before. It's about how lack of confidence almost destroyed my emotional energy, which in turn almost destroyed my ability to write. I write thrillers. There's usually some kind of military theme. Damn it, it takes me a long time to write them.

"My first three books were best-sellers. You never know how it happens, but you're grateful as hell when it does. It's just that after three best-sellers you think there are people out there who are going to buy your books. You start counting on it. So my fourth book, of course, was expected to sell very well, but the opposite happened. Reviewers liked it, which should've given me a warning right there. But you couldn't give the damn book away. It was a bomb. Nothing. You could hear the crickets chirping.

"It really got to me. I was scared. Maybe it was all over. I wrote my next book under a terrible sense of fear. It was painful. For the first time in my life I had to struggle to make myself work, like someone crawling out of bed in the morning after only a couple of hours' sleep. I'd been like a workman—nine o'clock in the morning, punch in, start writing. But now I was thinking I didn't have it anymore. You get all twisted around inside. You want to make it fresh, but then you're afraid of getting even further away from what made people like your stuff, then you remind yourself that they don't like your stuff. Or something. You've lost your confidence.

"There was this bad guy in the novel I was writing. One night I get up at three o'clock in the morning, go to my computer, and give this guy an eye patch, like a pirate. I go through the whole document, and everywhere the bad guy shows up I say something about his eye patch. Then

I just sit there staring at it. It was like I'd allowed myself to be completely humiliated because I was afraid. Now I'm reduced to putting corny eye patches on my villains. What next? Why not have him twirl his mustache? Maybe he should tie the heroine to some railroad tracks. I was just losing it.

"I couldn't go on that way. You just can't write without confidence. You can't do it. And here's this fickle audience that I don't understand. How can I build up my confidence by trying to please people when I don't know why they like what they like? I don't have any control over that. And what I saw was that I'd never had any control over that.

"That's when it hit me. You know, a lot of writers, what we do when we write is we're writing the book we want to read. We're writing to please ourselves. And I'm just an ordinary guy, so if I like it, you figure maybe other people will like it.

"That was the key. I had to go back to writing a book one guy would want to read—me. That I knew I could do.

"I started over. I scrapped the book I'd been working on. Suddenly the world was simple. There was one reader in the world, me, and I knew everything about how to make him happy. What can I say? Eight months later I had a book I liked. My editor liked it. And it sold. Thank God."

All writers face the problem of confidence. Take Hemingway. How did he give himself confidence during his prime? He too had to focus on something he could control. In his case, sentence by sentence he'd force himself to think about what he called "the next true thing." That helped him stay in the moment, which gave him the confidence and energy to keep on.

No matter who you are or what you're doing or why you're not feeling confident, there's something you can control that you can focus on, and then you will feel more confident.

Martin, 37: "Every time I hear some woman on television say there are no good men out there, I want to yell, '*I'm* a good guy. *I'm* out there.'

And there are lots of guys like me out there. But we're overlooked, because we're just good, solid, nice guys, and that's all.

"I got divorced at 29. I think my wife just got married too early, before she knew what she wanted. She said I was a great guy, but I didn't make her happy. She was unavailable emotionally. When I got mad, she said she couldn't deal with my anger. So she left.

"That really damaged my confidence because we had everything you need to make a relationship work. At least I thought so. But I picked up the pieces and tried starting over. It's a lot harder to meet women, though, once you've turned 30 and you're not so interested in going to clubs. I tried, and I either couldn't get women interested in me at all or we'd start going out and for one reason or another things wouldn't work out.

"I guess a lot of people fall into the mind-set I fell into. I'd be at some event and I'd see some woman and my very first thought would be that things wouldn't work out. I had no confidence in myself or the process or women or anything. I got to the point where I had so little emotional energy for dating that I didn't go out at all for over a year and a half.

"I'm embarrassed to tell you what sort of shocked me out of this. Early one Saturday evening I went to one of my local video stores and drifted back into the porn section. I was surprised at how crowded it was. Lonely guys in their thirties, forties, fifties, on up. And I looked at them and I thought, 'That's my future if I give up now.'

"I could accept that I didn't know how to find a wonderful woman who'd fall in love with me and become my wife and stay with me forever. That's a big prize. But one thing I knew absolutely for sure. I would never, ever find that woman in the porn section of my local video store.

"I was a lonely guy who I knew would be a good husband for someone. I could spend the rest of my life a lonely guy renting porn or I could spend the rest of my life trying to meet real women. At least if I tried, I'd have a chance. Who knows what would happen? But there are things you can do to meet women. You can go to dances. You can go to singles night at the museum. You can take out personal ads. You can join an organization that means something to you where you also might meet women. You can take classes. You can lose a few pounds and dress a little better.

"This is all stuff you have control over. This is all stuff you can do *excellently*. You can feel confident about writing an *excellent* personal ad. You can feel confident because you're learning to dance.

"I promised myself I was going to keep on trying until I was too old to try. I was never again going to worry about whether I'd ultimately find someone. Why should I make myself miserable thinking about a success I can't control when I can make myself happy doing things I do have control over?"

I almost don't want to tell you what happened because the whole point of this is that you can get confidence when you focus on processes you can control. I don't want you to think of this as a back-door route to success. Then you're thinking about outcomes again. And you're back in the trap.

On the other hand, it's a simple fact that confidence gives you *your only chance* at success. Did Martin find someone to love who would love him back? He did. At his church he joined a group of people who worked with people from other churches at rehabbing houses for the poor. One Saturday afternoon he found himself, hammer in hand, working alongside a shy dark-haired woman. They got to talking, found they agreed about a lot, started going out. Eventually they got married, and now they have three children.

On their fourth date, Martin learned that a few years before, this woman too had decided to let go of worrying about whether she found the right guy or not. The confidence that attracted Martin to her came from her feeling good about the process she was going through. They really were soul mates.

Confidence You Can Count On

The way you give yourself an emotional energy boost here is to focus on an area where your confidence has suffered. Then ask yourself what is one small thing you can do that you have absolute control over. Maybe you're facing a lot of tough competition at work, and maybe you're feeling far from the top of the heap. But what *can* you do? Can you come in an hour early from now on? Can you take a class to upgrade your skills? Is there someone you can ask for advice and mentoring? Can you just try to do better work?

There's always something you can do that's small enough so you can feel confident of your ability to do it. It doesn't matter what it is. The last thing you need to think about is finding the perfect step to rebuild your confidence. The most important thing is that you do something you have control over. Then your confidence will come back by itself. And you'll never lose emotional energy again.

24

Worry Is the Cracker Crumbs in the Bed of Life

Emotional Energy Booster #24

Worry is painful, but that's the least bad thing about it. Far worse is the way worry chews up your heart and mind and energy. Worries are psychological termites. Of course, when you worry you think you're *dealing* with things, but you're not. You're just suffering.

So it's time you put an end to worry, isn't it? Good. Because I have a plan that works. To help you understand, I want to show you something.

If Worry Is a Bed of Torment, What's the Mattress Made Of?

It's quarter to midnight. Out of the six billion people on this planet, let's focus in on three very different people in three very different places. Each is lying in bed alone, staring into the darkness. The first two are at peace. The last is racked with worry.

The first is an ordinary guy who works in an office. He has just gotten into bed and is about to settle into a long and restful sleep. Thinking about the day just passed and the day to come, he's not worried. There are problems to deal with, but even if things don't quite work out the way he'd like at work or at home, still he knows that everything will be okay.

The second man is a prisoner on death row scheduled for execution in the morning. He's lying in bed with his eyes wide open. But—and this might surprise you—he feels surprisingly calm too. Death is certain to come. He knows it'll be painless. He feels he's made his peace with God. In a strange but true way, he knows that everything will be okay, and that's a comfort.

But the third man is in utter torment. He too is scheduled for execution tomorrow. But his situation is different. He's in a foreign prison, facing death for a crime he didn't commit, although he can't prove it. He knows his lawyers and the United States government are working to try to get the head of state to pardon him. He knows they might succeed. But they might fail.

Now, if he really is going to die, he'll be in the same situation as the second man. Death will be quick. So in a sense everything will be okay. If he's released, he'll go back to living a life like the first man, and everything will be okay. Either way, he could find peace. People in either situation do find peace. But he doesn't know which fate will be his, so he's trapped in worry and torment.

You and Your Worry

Most of us go through our lives burdened like that third man. We know that in some way we're at a fork in the road. Either you'll get that great new job or you won't. Your marriage will work out or it won't. The stock market will go up this year or it won't. Many of us find that our lives are filled with uncertainty in many ways all at the same time. And so we carry around a horrible burden of worry.

Have you been wondering where your emotional energy has gone?

Check out how much you worry. You can have ...
the world, but worry will still exhaust you.

┌───┐
│   │
│   *Diagnostic Question #24*   │
│   │
│   *Would you say, "I worry a lot"?*   │
│   *A* **yes** *answer to this question means that this secret* │
│   *will give you a big boost of emotional energy.* │
│   │
└───┘

If you want to end worry, you have to understand what it's really all about. Many of us make a mistake. We think that worry is all about fear of something bad happening. But that's not true. Remember the second man, the one who knew he was going to die the next day? He wasn't worried. For sure, something bad was going to happen, but that's the point: He knew what was going to happen. And human beings' miraculous ability to cope made it possible for him to deal with that inevitable fate and get to the point where he could see that indeed everything would be okay.

So worry is not about something bad happening.

It's about *not knowing* what is going to happen.

And that's how we exhaust ourselves. Worry isn't fear. Worry is a kind of mindless scuttling around. It's not thinking, but just cycling over the same possibilities as we find ourselves compulsively playing out all the different alternatives.

To build up your emotional energy, you have to let go of worry. But of course, as you well know, you can't just tell yourself to stop worrying. You know what happens when a friend tells you to stop worrying. You tell your friend that she just doesn't understand everything you're having to deal with.

Climbing Out of the Worry Trap

When you're worrying you're saying, "I don't know how things are going to turn out, but I'm afraid they're going to turn out badly." Think about what you're really doing. You're focusing on the possible bad outcomes. If you're driving to the airport to catch a plane and you get caught in a traffic jam, you're going to focus on the possible bad outcome of missing your plane. If things get to the point where you know you're going to miss your plane, you're going to focus on the possible bad outcome of people being upset because you've missed your meeting.

It's as if worry is a probe that is constantly searching for the possible bad outcomes that lurk in your life. But there are always possible bad outcomes to everything. Maybe not likely. But possible. No wonder worry feeds on itself.

You can't deal with worries by killing them one at a time. In fact, because of worry's brilliance at turning up possible bad outcomes, your worry is going to make you feel that it's smarter than you are. That's how a lot of us go through life. "Of course, I'm just a big fat idiot, but my worry is a genius. It's always coming up with issues I never would've thought of."

Because your worry has convinced you that it's smarter than you are, you let it take over. And a lot of the people who loved you, like your parents, worried about you as a way of showing their love. So you let worry take over as a way of your showing your love for yourself. On the job a lot of us are rewarded highly for being professional worriers. So we let worry take over in the hope that it will be a talisman for success.

Meanwhile, we know for sure that worry torments us, exhausts us, and does absolutely nothing good for us. Worry never comes up with good ideas. It never yields comfort. It never brings your ship to any safe harbor.

If worry is your way of constantly thinking about how things are going to turn out badly, *the only way to replace it is with thoughts about how in the end, one way or another, everything's going to be okay.* Maybe everything won't be perfect. Maybe things won't turn out exactly the way you wanted. But really, if you look deeply into any of the alternatives you're facing, you'll see that you'll be okay, your life will turn out okay, and just maybe everything will be for the best.

Let me make clear exactly what I'm saying. Worry isn't something that happens to you. Worry is something you do. Worry is thinking about bad outcomes. But because it's something you do, you can do something different. If you can think about warthogs, you can also think about puppies. If you can think about bad things happening, you can instead think about good things happening or about how the things that will happen will be for the good. The very fact that you have the capacity for worry means that you have the capacity for thinking about the future, and that means that you have the capacity for searching through your future to find good things, not bad things.

No one ever, *ever* looked back on his life and wished he'd spent more time worrying. Almost everyone looks back and regrets the time they've spent worrying. What people do wish they'd done is spend more time thinking about how everything will be okay and then doing things to make that happen.

Even chronic worriers discover that they're able to switch over to trying to think about how everything will be okay. This is nothing more than a new habit of mind. That's all worry is: a bad habit of mind.

Here's the most straightforward way to do this. Take a situation you're worried about. It could be anything. Now ask yourself, "How can I look at this *in a more positive way*?" There's always an angle or a perspective on a situation you're worried about from which you can realistically say that things will be okay.

Skeptical? Ninety percent of the people who are emotionally exhausted by worry have never even *tried* to think about how everything will be okay. I challenge you to try this for one week. Take it one day at a time for seven days. And on each one of those days whenever you start worrying, *make* yourself focus on how everything will be okay no matter what happens. That means listing all the ways things will be okay. At least think about how things won't be so bad. How maybe things will be better than you think.

Let's say you're worried about your relationship. Look, if it's really bad, you'll be a lot happier on your own. And so in that way things will be okay. Or it will get better and you'll stay. Just because you're panicking about how things can turn out doesn't mean you can't feel safe when you actually look at the alternatives you're facing.

Maybe what you think is bad is really good. You're worried about getting fired. Well, perhaps you don't have to be afraid because being fired is an opportunity to make changes in your career or in where you live that actually will lead you in a better direction.

Maybe you can fix things and make them turn out better. Suppose you're worried about a downturn in the economy and how it will affect your small business. But perhaps things will be okay if you can cut costs, market more aggressively, and focus in on a more profitable product line.

Maybe you can step back, look at the bigger picture, lengthen your time horizon, and let go of the tiny, narrow, specific little future you've pinned your hopes on. From some broader or different perspective, truly everything will be okay. Instead of spending your energy worrying, spend your energy finding that perspective. Anyone can do this.

Mark, 32: "I'll tell you the way I felt. It was like being at the bottom of a deep, dark well. That's how bad I was sunk in worry. And you can't even talk about figuring a way out because when you're at the bottom of the well and you look up you don't see anything that you can use to help yourself figure a way out. You look and there's nothing.

"I was working for this big high-tech company when high-tech manufacturing crashed. Right after the Internet boom crashed. People were being laid off left and right. So I'm thinking I'm going to be laid off too and . . . well, just doomed. I was like, 'Oh, my God, I won't have any income, I won't have a job, I won't be able to find a job.'

"I got into the stupidest fight with my girlfriend, but it saved me. I was telling her how worried I was and she said, like people do, 'Everything's going to be okay.' I said, 'Don't give me that crap.' We started going back and forth like kids. Everything's going to be okay. Everything's *not* going to be okay. We were really yelling. Finally I said, 'How is everything going to be okay?'

"She really surprised me. She was so wise. She said, 'Look, eventually you'll find a job. It might take a little longer or it might happen faster than you think. And who really knows whether longer or faster is better? Your new job might seem a little better or a little worse. You might go through a rough patch. People do. But who really knows what's best in the long run? In any case, you'll eventually get a new job and everything will be okay.'

"I was like, 'Well, when you put it like that . . .' That was it. She took my worry away. What I was worrying about was *details*. Maybe some of them wouldn't be okay. But in the long run, I didn't need to be afraid.

"We'd both been thinking about my future. But I was just focusing on the dark parts. She was focusing on the positive parts. We were both spending energy thinking. I was exhausting myself from where I was spending my energy. She got energy from where she spent hers. So why not do what she did? It's all just thinking about stuff. Why not make it work for you?"

Worry is like eating potato chips. Once you start going, it's hard to stop. Yet people stop all the time. And you will stop when you find a way, like Mark did (with a little help), to step back and put a little of that wonderful brainpower of yours into thinking about how things will work out fine. If at first you try and don't succeed, step around to the side a little bit. Find the right distance and the right angle, and you'll see that worry is silly.

Worry Is Always Optional, and It's Always a Bad Option

You say it's Pollyannaish to believe that worry is silly? Sure it is, from the point of view of troubleshooting. That's what troubleshooters do: They look for all the ways things might go wrong. They are hired worriers. We need them to be hypervigilant. But worry is sheer poison for your vitality. It does nothing but suck the life out of you.

Who's happy in this world we live in? Who accomplishes big things?

Who gets involved in really interesting activities? Who develops their talents? Who finds love? Who realizes their potential? Only people who make their emotional energy a priority. Worriers piss it all away.

There is a time and place for troubleshooting, no question about it. But your need for more emotional energy must rule. And to get that you have to be able to find a way to see that there's nothing to be afraid of. And there always is a way.

Margaret, 42: "Most people worry about getting cancer. But what do you do after you *know* you're going to die of cancer? That's what happened to me. It's what we all dread. The doctor tells you you've got such-and-such cancer, and I'm a nurse. I knew it was fatal. Of course it hits you hard. You cry. You're angry. Of course you're scared. But at some point it hits you that you're not going to die tomorrow or even next week. What's really ahead of you is *life.* Maybe not as much of it as some people have, but you have it. Plus you have all the people who are in your life. So what are you going to do about this life that you have? Are you going to screw it up?

"I have a husband and children ages seven and nine. Of course I'm worried about them. They're worried about me. But you've got to believe me when I tell you that worry is not the way to spend your last months on earth with the people you love.

"Here's what I did. Believe me, we all need as much emotional energy as we can give each other. So instead of thinking about all the bad things that could happen to us in the future, we think about all the good things that can happen. For example, my children are going to lose their mother. It makes me cry just to say this. But I'm not worried anymore. Instead of thinking about how they're going to lose me, I think about how they're going to know I was an important part of their lives. I think about the fact that they will remember me and about the good things they will remember about me.

"And I could worry about how they'll turn out, but even if I lived to ninety I could still worry about my kids. But instead I think about what kind of kids they are, and I imagine them having good lives and finding things they love in life and having families of their own. I imagine them giving their own kids the good things they've gotten from me.

"I don't know. I mean, you can think about the good things or you can think about the bad things. But you'll never stop thinking about the bad things until you look for good things to think about. And then things change. It's not just about what's in your head. Your life is different.

"For example, for some crazy reason I started worrying about my children's birthdays. My husband's not the kind of guy who does parties really well. So then I thought, 'What's the opposite of worry here?' Well, come on, everyone I know is going to want my kids to have happy birthdays. They're going to have happy birthdays. And you see, I just know it was thinking about good things like that that gave me the idea of making video birthday cards for each child for each of their birthdays until they reached twenty-one. It just made me so happy to think about doing this for them."

Because this woman thinks about how her family will be all right, she can *see* how they will be all right. This is a person who really understands the importance of nourishing your emotional energy.

Mastering the Art of Peace of Mind

Here are the three ingredients for finding the perspective that will make it possible for you to see that everything will be okay. Master these, and you'll have mastered the secrets of peace of mind.

The first ingredient is *patient timing*. A lot of worry gets taken up with thinking about when something is going to happen. You want a good new job, but you press the panic button because you're invested in finding that great new job in the next month or two.

Worry about death itself is an issue of timing. We all know we're going to die. Why destroy the quality of your life tonight by making a big deal about exactly when you're going to die? Look at it like this. Who can say when the perfect time to die is? Almost all of us die either too soon or too late. We'd like to live a long time, but if you had to choose, maybe you'd say it's better to die too soon than too late. Who wants to hang on so long that the quality of life is lousy and the last thoughts people have of you are you at your worst? So what's there to be afraid of? Not knowing how things are going to turn out for the people you care about? You'd have to live about 150 years to get the whole story on how your grandchildren's lives turn out, and then there'd be great-great-grandchildren's lives to worry about.

Think about some worry of yours and think about how impatience or some arbitrary idea about when something is supposed to happen is forcing you to worry. But if you let go of the timing issue, fear disappears and you can let go of worry. Instead, you can put energy into thinking about the good things that can happen, regardless of when exactly that will be.

The second ingredient is *being open to a whole spectrum of outcomes*. Where we go wrong is getting hung up on wanting one tiny particular outcome. We started doing this as kids. Walk into any supermarket and some kid is having a total fit because his health-conscious mother won't buy him Count Chocula. There are a million different cereals. He goes nuts because he can't have that *one*.

Cut to our adult selves and you find . . . no difference. Let's say you're dating someone and you know he's feeling iffy about you. You're terribly afraid he's going to dump you. You lie awake at night in an agony of worry, just like that third man we talked about earlier who didn't know if he'd live or die. And you go through all that worry because that man you're involved with is your Count Chocula. It's him or nothing. Him or the abyss. You're afraid because you've set it up so that there's only one way things can be okay.

But if you say to yourself, "How can I look at this differently?" then you start realizing that there are a lot of fish in the sea. Not just when it comes to relationships, but when it comes to all the opportunities we care about. And how can you know beforehand what's best? A little humility about our ability to see into the future helps an awful lot in letting go of that one particular outcome you were hoping for. Neither you nor I are that smart. There are, in fact, many ways good and wonderful things can happen to us. Many of these will be a complete surprise. And that makes it easy to think that everything will be okay.

The third ingredient is *trusting your ability to cope*. I know, you and I can look back and point to more than one incident that casts doubt on our ability to cope. We panicked and screwed up. But so what? As they used to say on *Sesame Street,* everyone makes mistakes, oh yes they do! But our mistakes don't invalidate the fact that we can cope. We make bad decisions, but then we go on to make good decisions. We get knocked down, but then we pick ourselves up. We're stupid, but then we get smart.

The most important truth about people is that we *can* cope. All of us. Nothing has ever happened in human history that people couldn't find a way to cope with. Inside we may feel fearful and miserable, so inside we give ourselves the message that we're not coping. But don't confuse those feelings with the reality of your ability to rise to the occasion.

> *Emotional energy booster #24*
> *End worry by not thinking about how things*
> *might go wrong; instead start thinking about*
> *all the ways things will be okay.*

Don't Just Stew There, Do Something

Here's something that will help. *Action is the antidote to worry.* Your mind can tell you things will be okay, but help yourself further by taking a specific action to deal with whatever it is you're worried about every time you worry. If you find you're worrying, get up and do something. Don't fret, act. *It doesn't matter what you do* as long as it has even a small chance of bringing you one step closer to coping with your problem.

Are you lying in bed at night worrying? Get out of bed, and if you can do nothing else, write down a to-do list. Even that's an action. You'll see how action diminishes worry.

Suppose that every time you worry you do *one* thing, anything, as long as it's constructive. That way you build a relationship of trust with yourself. You're saying to yourself, "Self, I take care of you. I won't let you stew. I'll do things to help." *And your self will stop worrying when it sees that you're there to do things to take care of it.*

25

The More You Give, the More You Get

Emotional Energy Booster #25

Imagine a magic bottle of wine. Every time you pour out a glassful, the bottle fills up again. The faster you pour, the more quickly it fills up. But this gets even better. The more wine you pour from this magic bottle, the better the wine itself gets. So if you own one of these magic bottles and want more and better wine, the best thing to do is to give as much of it away as possible. The more you give, the more you'll get.

Emotional energy is magic too. I mean that quite literally. It has magical properties. And the most magical of its properties is the fact that the more energy you give, the more energy you get.

Sam, 41: "People look at me and think I have it made because I'm a good-looking guy with a really interesting career. Yeah, but things aren't as easy for me as people think. I own this small biotech company, and I'm supposed to keep getting positive results from the new drugs we design. But sometimes you work really hard and you hit a losing streak. People in the industry look at you like you have a bad smell. I've recently gone through one of these streaks. Then my wife and I broke up. People think I landed on my feet, but I loved Caitlin and I was heartbroken when she decided she wasn't getting what she needed from me.

"When my marriage ended it was a really bad time for me. I don't know how to describe it. It's as if my world had been in color and it suddenly started coming in in black and white. There was no joy left. I was written up as one of the top eligible bachelors in town and it didn't matter to me. How do you put the fizz back in the seltzer when it's gone?

"A guy in my company, an older scientist, kind of my mentor, took me aside one day and said he noticed there was something wrong. We went out for drinks and started talking. Finally he told me something shocking. He told me that the biggest thing wrong with me was that I wasn't as good a guy as I thought I was. I was selfish and spoiled. That's why Caitlin broke up with me, he said. And it was time for me to do something about it. 'Be a good person and it will save your life,' he said. 'You're single again. If you just hang out there like the playboy you've been, you'll attract the kind of women you deserve. You'll get taken again and again. But if you do something really good, it will scare away the bad women, and it will scare away all the bad karma you've been building up in this incredibly lucky life of yours.'

"I didn't know what to do, but for some reason the idea of giving back had always been in my head. You know, helping people who didn't have some of the luck or advantages I had. So I decided, Hey, I'll be a Big Brother. I'll help one kid who really needs it. You know, it's not going to save the world. But it might save one kid.

"So I signed up, went through the interviews, had to wait to get a kid assigned to me. But all that just made me feel more strongly that I needed to do this. And it's the best thing I've ever done. It changes the equation of my life. It makes me feel I'm a person of substance, someone with something to give, and I'm not a fraud, because I do give. I could just write a check, but that really wouldn't mean anything. You've got to do it with your whole soul. Give what's really precious, your time. All I know is that since I've been involved with this my energy and my spirits have lifted."

The emotional energy inside you makes *you* one of those magic wine bottles yourself, the way it did with Sam.

Diagnostic Question #25

Are you feeling low, drained, bitter, and flat these days, as if you've broken up with someone you love?

*A **yes** answer to this question means that this secret will give you a big boost of emotional energy.*

You may feel empty. I understand. That's a way people with low emotional energy commonly feel. But you're not empty. Your emotional energy isn't gone. It never is. That's where the miracle of emotional resilience comes from. You just haven't been tapping in to it. Now you can see how different emotional energy is from physical energy. With physical energy you have to get it to be able to give it. With emotional energy, magically, you can get it *by* giving it.

Emotional energy booster #25
The most magical way to get emotional energy is by giving it:
showing your love for the world one person at a time,
one patch of ground at a time.

The Magic of Giving

Now, you might wonder how this secret works. There are two reasons why it's so powerful.

When you tap into your own capacity for generosity, kindness, and goodness, you immediately feel better about yourself as a person. It's the fastest, most powerful way to do for your insides what fantastic new clothes would do for your outsides. You've done something that a moment earlier might have felt impossible, and yet you've now proved it's easy. You've shown yourself that the fire still burns within you, and that means you've taught yourself a deep and powerful lesson about your depth of resilience.

Second, when you love the world, it loves you back. Think of it as good karma. But merely having a vague attitude of love toward the world doesn't count. You have to do specific, positive things, like the ones I'm going to outline in a moment. And you have to keep doing them even when it feels pointless—*especially* when it feels pointless. You may or may not immediately get back what you give. But sooner or later you will get back much more than you gave.

How to Get Energy by Giving Love

No act of love and kindness is too small to do or too big to dream of doing. Think big, think small, think everything in between. But make it personal and specific. You could simply think about helping someone who really needs it. But here are some even easier suggestions, based on what high-energy people report worked best as a way to plug in to love and get back a big bonus of emotional energy.

Be more affectionate. I guarantee that the people you care about are missing your affection. We forget to be affectionate. We let it slide. The more emotionally fatigued you are, the more likely you are to stop being affectionate. But when you show affection, you'll get a big boost in energy. You say you're already an affectionate person? I'm not saying you're not. But you're probably not showing as much affection as you think. And the people around you are probably used to the level of affection you do show. Wherever you're starting from, showing more affection will give you more energy.

Have a be-nice-to-everyone day. Get up in the morning and make it your fixed goal to be especially warm to everyone you encounter. Maybe in general you think you're already nice to people. Be a little nicer. Maybe you recognize that you're generally brusque or detached. Astound everyone by showing your friendliness and concern.

Ask everyone you meet, "How are you?" as if you really want to know, and then listen to what they have to say. Ask follow-up questions. If they just say, "Fine," say, "Are you sure everything's okay?" Be *there* for the other person and what they're going through.

Listen to someone you don't want to listen to. Too often the people we share our lives with blame, complain, and go on and on about stuff we don't really care about. That means that too often we go through our days giving off a please-just-shut-up vibe. Well, if everyone is telling everyone else to shut up, everyone is feeling invisible and silenced. Everyone is feeling desperate to be heard. So you be the one to do the hearing. Let people get things off their chest in your presence. It doesn't require more than asking a question and listening to the answer. Even if you think the other person is wrong, listen anyway. The emotional energy of the world will be healed far better and faster by people feeling heard than by people being right.

Smile. What's more powerful than a toddler's smile? There you have it: proof that you don't need the wattage of a Julia Roberts or a Tom Cruise to turn the world. You just need to smile more often. Ask yourself this: When you see the person you love first thing in the morning, do you smile? You should know that every time you don't smile when you see the person you love first thing in the morning, you're sucking just a little energy out of your relationship. That's the point. Every time you smile when you might not have smiled before, you make the world a warmer, happier place.

Help someone. Make it real, concrete, experiential. Start with the people you're closest to. Give them something they've wanted that you've always said you can't give them. Or ask them if there's anything they need from you. Give them a massage, run an errand for them, listen to them. Then spread your circle of help. Be helpful to people you work with. Go through an entire workday asking yourself what you would do if your goal were to be helpful rather than efficient.

Show that you appreciate the people in your life. I'm not talking about flattery. I'm talking about sincerely appreciating people for who they are and what they do. And people feel most appreciated when you express how grateful you feel. The key is to demonstrate that you're not taking the person for granted. And it's amazing how much emotional energy you generate when you do this. Most of us are caught in a trap where we don't give because we don't feel given to. Sometimes it seems as though the world is filled with people standing around with arms folded. But you can break that cycle. If you appreciate people for what they do, they feel given to, and then they give to you and to others. What goes around comes around, so why not have the stuff that goes around be good stuff?

Every day, before you start out, ask yourself, "How can I be a better person today?" Any answer will do. Then act on it. We all have little goals for ourselves every day—to eat less, to exercise more, to work harder, to work less. But how often do we start out with being kinder as our goal for the day? Just make your first and primary goal to do one simple thing to be a better, kinder person than you were the day before.

APPENDIX
The *Physical* Energy Factor

❋

The average person living in a developed country is lucky. His diet and lifestyle give him lots of physical energy. It's emotional energy that's typically in shortest supply.

Still, if you've been in a "Why don't I have more energy?" state, there is the possibility that there's something wrong on the physical energy side of the equation. I want to help you make sure you're doing everything sensible to build up your physical energy. I've consulted with leading experts on the causes of physical fatigue. So if you think you may need more physical energy, here's what to do.

The Best Things to Do for More Physical Energy

Forget fads. Forget gimmicks. Here's the real story, the real inside dope. If you're serious about having more energy, here's what high-energy people actually do to take care of the physical side of the equation.

Get more sleep. This is the number-one reason people don't have more physical energy. Nowhere do smart people behave more stupidly. Some people say it's not possible to get more sleep. They think energy experts are crazy: "If you knew my schedule, you'd know it was ridiculous to think that I could get more sleep." But just the way budget experts can show people who "can't save" how in fact they can cut back on their expenses, you can get more sleep if you make it a priority. If you don't get enough sleep, don't complain about being tired. The only correct way to think of it is that sleep is fuel, and you need to get the sleep fuel that you need. Any less than that, and you're running on empty.

What to do: You must determine how much sleep you need to live without fatigue. Everyone's different, but the overwhelming majority of people (and why should you be an exception?) need more sleep than they're getting. If you're saying you only need six hours, you're saying, "I'm a very, very special person." Maybe your soul is, but physiologically? I doubt it. So if you're physically tired, do this. For the next couple of nights set your alarm so that you get ten hours of sleep. Go to bed earlier if you have to. Then see how you feel. Then for a couple of nights set your alarm so that you get nine and a half hours sleep. Again see how you feel. It's almost certain that you'll notice you're feeling a lot more energy. Cut back half an hour at a time until you notice you're feeling less than optimal energy. Then go back and *add* half an hour to your nightly sleep budget. That's the amount of sleep you need. It will almost certainly be more than you're getting now.

Exercise. Everyone needs exercise. Twenty minutes of fairly intensive exercise almost every day makes a huge difference in how energetic people feel. There's something about the way the body works that means that you have to put out a certain amount of physical energy to feel even more physical energy.

What to do: "I'm too busy." "I don't like to exercise." Guess what? Most people who exercise feel that way. But they know the importance of exercise. The key is finding the same time every day and then making it a part of your daily routine. And most people who exercise don't like to feel pain or boredom any more than you do. What they do is make sure they find something they like, or hate least. Or they do what they have to do to make it enjoyable (like watching TV while on the treadmill). Or they just do it. Here are some things you might want to try: jumping rope, dancing, cardio boxing, squash, swimming. The point is to get your heart and body moving at a faster rate for a good twenty minutes every day.

Eliminate caffeine after your morning coffee. There was a surprising consensus about how important this is. The later in the day you take in caffeine, the more tired you end up feeling.

What to do: It's okay to have a cup or two of coffee in the morning, before work or when you first get to the office. But that's it. And make sure you're not taking in caffeine via cola drinks. If you're feeling tired in the middle of the day, caffeine is not the solution. It's part of the problem. You need more sleep, more exercise, or a better diet.

Eat a balanced diet. With so many fad diets around, it's not cool to tell people they need to eat a balanced diet. There's only one thing, though. It's true. A diet well balanced among protein, complex carbohydrates, and a small amount of healthy fat is the single best source of energy from food.

What to do: You can make it complicated or simple. I prefer simple. Whenever you eat, make sure there's some protein, some carbohydrates (I'm talking about whole-grain products, fruits, and vegetables), and a little fat. If you just do that, you'll be doing better than most people.

Take vitamins. There's a lot of hype and controversy when it comes to vitamins. But do what the smartest, the most knowledgeable, and most sensible experts recommend.

What to do: Take a good multiple vitamin with a meal daily. Make sure it's a pill that has all the vitamins and minerals. You don't need to take a lot of pills—simply take the vitamin pill with the most stuff in it. Go to your local drugstore and ask your pharmacist to recommend the most complete vitamin pill on the shelf for someone of your age and gender. If you have special health needs—whether you're pregnant, ill, or something else—ask your doctor if there are special vitamins that are necessary for you.

Reduce sugar. Candy bar commercials notwithstanding, sugar in any form sets you up for an energy crash.

What to do: You don't have to eliminate desserts and sweets from your life. But you do have to eliminate them from the times of your day when you want to feel energetic. And if you suddenly feel weak and hungry, eat a piece of fruit or have a light, healthy meal.

Drink water. A surprising number of people feel fatigue because they're dehydrated, and not just in hot weather either.

What to do: You have to make drinking water a habit. People have different tricks. They always stop when they pass a water fountain and take some sips. They carry a bottle of water around with them and make sure they finish at least one bottle every day. They ask for water every time they eat out and make sure to drink it. But however you do it, drink at least eight big glasses of water a day.

Stop eating three hours before you go to bed. At night you have to give your body a rest from everything, and that includes digestion. Dealing with a lot of food just before sleep puts a load on your body. Plus, dealing with all that food can make your sleep restless and interrupted.

What to do: In the evening, know when you're going to go to bed. Then plan your evening so that you finish your last bite of food three hours before your bedtime. The one slight exception to this is the very small amount of complex carbohydrates—no more than one slice of bread or a couple of cookies or crackers—that you may eat just before bed to help you fall asleep.

Don't drink alcohol before sleep. Wine, beer, or any other alcoholic beverage shouldn't be used as a nightcap or a way to relax before sleep. If you drink before you go to sleep, when the alcohol wears off, it tends to wake you up, producing interrupted sleep.

What to do: As with eating, have your last drink of alcohol at least three hours before you go to bed.

I was very interested in discovering whether there were any special "secret" ways to get a supercharge of physical energy. I asked my specialists what they would recommend if someone came to them and said the following: "I'm a fairly high-energy person, and I take good care of myself. But I've just been elected president of the United States and I need extra energy. What can I do?"

The answer might surprise you. *There are no backdoor ways to extra physical energy*. The only way to get the highest possible level of physical energy is to do everything on the list I've just given you. Special energy drinks and bars? They're useless at best, often lower your energy, and are in many cases dangerous because they contain harmful substances. Beware of tricks and gimmicks. The physical route to high energy consists in doing the basics. Now you know what they are.

Special Problems

What if you're doing all these things and you're still feeling physically tired? Then you should see your doctor. You should also see your doctor if you suspect there might be a reason for your feeling tired other than just not doing everything you need to do to take care of yourself.

Believe it or not, when I asked a number of prominent physicians whom they would go to see if they suddenly found themselves feeling unusually tired for a long period of time, they all said they'd see their internist.

Most internists are in a sense physical energy specialists. They have to be. "Doctor, I feel tired all the time" is the most common complaint people bring to them. And a good internist takes this seriously. That's because fatigue can *sometimes* (but only sometimes) be a sign of a serious underlying condition. And if you've been unusually tired, you have to rule out the possibility that your thyroid, kidneys, liver, autoimmune system, or digestive system have something wrong with them. There are scores of diseases and conditions that make people unusually tired. You should rule out the possibility that you have one of these.

Since many people worry about cancer, let me point out that most cancers don't have fatigue as an early warning sign.

Another physical condition that people worry about when they're feeling tired is chronic fatigue syndrome. This is a controversial diagnosis. I've talked to some of the leading experts, and here's what the current consensus seems to be.

Chronic fatigue syndrome is real. We may not know exactly what causes it or how to cure it, but if you have it, it's not just in your head.

But it's overwhelmingly likely that you don't have chronic fatigue syndrome. How can I say that? Because in fact it's quite rare. To qualify for the diagnosis, you have to pass through some rigid screens. First, you have to be extremely tired, so much so that you're virtually unable to function. Second, you have to rule out every other medical explanation for your fatigue. This takes months and requires going through many tests. Third, current diagnostic criteria require that serious, debilitating fatigue has to have lasted more than six months for chronic fatigue syndrome to be a possibility. If there is something wrong with you medically, it's probably not chronic fatigue syndrome.

If your doctor calls you into the office after you've had some tests to tell you about some condition you might have, a lot of important information is going to come at you in a short period of time. This is why it helps to bring a friend or relative with a clear head who can ask questions you might not think of and who can explain to you later some points you might have missed. Bring a pen and pad, and make sure you don't leave the office until you've gotten an answer to all your questions. If there's a reason why you might have trouble doing anything the doctor prescribes, talk to her about it.

Don't be embarrassed to call back if you have any further questions. If you find that something isn't working or is giving you side effects, talk to your doctor about that too. Above all, be active, and take responsibility for doing everything your doctor tells you to do.

The good news is that your doctor will probably find that there's nothing physically wrong with you. You're just pushing yourself too hard, you're neglecting the basics, *and you're doing nothing to build up your emotional energy.* And if there does happen to be something wrong with you, usually you can be made to feel a lot better, if not cured.

INDEX